THE DIARIES OF A PERSONAL TRAINER

by Nigel Taylor

INTRODUCTION

Hello and welcome to my book "The Diaries of a personal trainer." My name is Nigel Taylor and I'm a personal trainer, and have been as far back as I can remember. Whether it be part time or full time, un-certified or certified, training personal friends or training business clients it's always something I've done and enjoyed doing in some kind of fashion or other.

I was born and raised in the north of England by really great parents, the best anyone could wish for really. At school I was always really very thin and really very weak, but always seemed kind of popular with all the other kids, I got along with everyone, even the bullies left me alone, not that they were scared of me of course, but rather I guess they just didn't see me as any kind of threat which was just as well really as I couldn't fight my way out of a wet paper bag back then!

Thin as I may have been, I could put away some serious food though, but never put any weight on at all. Hardly surprising really though with a very fast metabolism and also considering I was very active playing soccer every night for hours and hours I wasn't very likely to put on any weight. In fact when I left school I was all of 140lb!

So, something had to change as I prepared myself for working life, and it did big time! I discovered lifting weights-long before I discovered beer-and promptly put on 60lb of muscle over the next two years, it was life changing, and it was my thing. Here`s my story….

MY LIFETIME OF FITNESS

HOW IT ALL BEGAN

One typically cold and rainy night in Chesterfield England way back in 1980, I was feeling very bored flicking through the only three TV channels we had back then BBC1, BBC2 & ITV-long before the days of cable and satellite-hoping to find something entertaining when a documentary called `Pumping Iron` came on. Not knowing anything about this I decided it may be worth watching.

So I settled down for the night and started watching, and was completely shocked by the size of these monsters filling my small TV screen, after about 15 minutes I realized these were real people and not some camera or computer enhanced figures. Right from that moment I knew I was destined to become a `Gym Rat` for life! Immediately after the show ended I called my friend who had also been watching equally impressed.

"Did you see the size of that guy? and what about that Arnold character with the weird last name?" we both agreed on a time and set off the next morning to a sports store in the local town center to purchase a cheap weight set of plastic sand filled weights, well they seemed good at the time. In our eagerness we hadn`t considered how we were to get them home. Since neither of us could drive at that time we had to walk the 5 miles home carrying a 100lb weights set! After a few very hard & long hours we finally got them home by which time we were both so tired and sore we didn`t start working out for another week! And that`s how it all began.

ACHES AND PAINS, AND EVEN MORE ACHES AND PAINS!

So, six months later I'm training like crazy, seven days a week sometimes twice a day. Constantly waking up the next morning unable to move because I'm so sore through over training No-Pain-No-Gain right? I'm quite proud of the fact that I'm able to get rid of the soreness each day just in time to hit the weights again.

No thought to any kind of diet, eating everything in sight and drinking lots of beer at the weekends, dressed in muscle shirts everywhere I go showing off those tiny biceps to anyone who is crazy enough to look!

Of course I'm not making any gains and have no idea why, but by now I'm totally obsessed with the weights, like a drug I must have my fix of iron. Yes! I have now progressed from the plastic sand filled ones to real iron weights. No! I didn't walk home 5 miles with these, I ordered them from a catalog along with a lightweight bench, all of which was delivered to the house.

I'm working out in the kitchen now which has turned into my gym with dad spotting me on a 150lb. bench press, this is getting hard work as dad isn't sure he can lift this, and come to think of it I'm not sure I can either!

Now this really isn't an ideal situation to have to carry all the equipment from a closet, set up the bench and all the weights which is a workout in itself. Work out, then put them all back again in the closet afterwards, and all the time we are keeping mom out of her kitchen. This goes on for a further two years with very little gains to show for my efforts, and then I finally see the light, I really need to join a gym.

ATTENDING MY FIRST REAL GYM

Around this time I happened to bump into an old school friend who I'd lost touch with over the years, he was also into lifting weights, and told me about this local gym he had found. So he said he`d take me down there to meet the owner if I wanted, I accepted his offer and eagerly awaited the next day when we arranged to go and check this gym out.

It was love at first sight! This is great, a real gym with real bodybuilders working out there. In fact it's an old Doctor`s surgery that someone has turned into a gym with very old equipment, some of which is homemade. The gym has no name and comes complete with a hole in the roof above the leg press machine. Now winter in England is no joke as its freezing and always seems to be snowing on leg day, and each time I emerge from the leg press I'm covered in snow! I love this place, it has real character and I'm still working out almost every day with of course no gains to show for my pains, plenty of pains at this point though, that's for sure!

One day I get lucky and meet the owner, a real genuinely great guy who informs me I'm over training and need to cut back to three sessions a week if I really want to develop muscle and strength, and also pay attention to my diet. I never considered I was doing too much and being a `gym addict` now I'm worrying about what I will do on my four days off.

But I take his word for it and do as he says, and like magic I start developing muscles without the previous pain, now I'm experiencing a nice soreness that isn't as severe as before. I'm getting to train with lots of experienced people now all offering great advice, and I'm in the best shape since I started and start to realize the mistakes I made in the beginning.

Two years later the owner moved to another part of town and opened a fantastic gym! This place has much more modern equipment, bigger building, a name and no holes in the roof! And is still going strong today. On my four days off I'm studying about various aspects of everything associated with the gym, correct form, nutrition, cardio etc. By this time it`s four years since I first started working out. I have a great training program, and for the first time I really know what I'm doing in a gym, in fact to the extent that I'm now a certified personal trainer. Certified under the gym I'm working at, at this time being certified under a nationally recognized organization hadn't really been thought of. That came later.

So the next few years are spent helping people in the gym with their fitness and nutrition etc. mostly part time in the evenings and weekends, more of a hobby than profession at this stage, but the good thing was I was learning all the time from people who ate, drank and breathed the gym world! It was a very infectious environment, and I thrived on it.

MARTIAL ARTS

Also, around this time a co-worker introduced me to Ju-Jitsu and kickboxing, which I immediately took to. As all kids growing up in England in the 70`s I was heavily into the Bruce Lee movies and wanted to be like him, with no kung-Fu classes available around that time I tried Karate, but after trying a few Karate lessons it just wasn't my thing, no disrespect to that form of martial arts but walking up and down a room punching and kicking wasn't exactly too thrilling, and certainly wasn't going to hold the attention of a young kid for very long.

Now Ju-Jitsu on the other hand, proved to be very exciting with all the throws, locks, chokes etc. I was hooked after the very first class. I started out at three lessons per week and with lots of private tuition from my friend who was already a black belt, so I very quickly advanced through the belts, after 10 years I'm a 3rd degree black belt myself.

This was Japanese Ju-Jitsu by the way, not the Brazilian version that became so popular in cage fighting later on. This was purely self-defense and extremely violent! They taught you to win no matter what!

Also twice a week I was kickboxing too, not the actually fighting but rather the training, I think it's fair to say I was in the best shape of my life at this time.

UNITED STATES HERE I COME!

So, onto the present day, I have now swapped the cold weather in England for the hot weather in South Texas! I never really felt settled in England, what with all that rain and cold and always envisioned myself moving somewhere hot. When the company I'd been working at for 10 years suddenly lost a major order they asked people to consider taking a voluntary lay off, the severance package they offered me was too good to turn down, so this was my big chance to make a fresh start somewhere else, and of course somewhere hot.

After careful research Texas seemed to be the ideal choice, with a reasonably good cost of living, and very hot weather this was for me. I started off in San Antonio, because of the Alamo! Seemed as good a place to start as any, which looks nothing like you see on the old movies nowadays. Then moved to Austin and then Round Rock where I am now.

Anyway, after starting off doing several crappy jobs I thought maybe it's time to try personal training full time, slight difference here as you must be certified by a nationally recognized organization, which basically means more money to pay to get started, but I figured it would get me a training job anywhere so would be a good investment.

MY FIRST PERSONAL TRAINING JOB .....USA STYLE!

So, after several weeks of studying for my personal training certification around the regular jobs I was doing at the time, I had now officially passed the exam, and was now recognized by one of the big name training certification organizations. With certificate in hand I set about finding a gym to work at. With so many gyms around these days, shouldn't be a problem. I applied at one of the big name gyms and was hired immediately. Sadly, it wasn't to be a good experience.

My first taste of being a full time personal trainer in one of the big corporate gyms in the United States lasted all of one day! I was excited to start training people but soon realized their philosophy is more to do with sales than genuinely helping people. Without doubt a case of purely money making and nothing more.

My first red flag concerning this place was during orientation, a two hour briefing about the company, and about personal training that was hosted by the head of human resources, nothing unusual about that of course, but the fact this lady was at least 80lb over weight was kind of shocking to say the least. She admitted she didn't work out, and proved her ignorance on several occasions by stating facts that clearly were not true about training! It was very obvious everyone in attendance knew she was wrong but no one felt like it was their job to correct her, after all, everyone wants to create a good first impression, and telling the head of human resources that's she's wrong might not go down too well.

Before I could be let loose to train clients they gave me two weeks of training, which was basically nothing more than sales training, after which I felt more equipped to be selling cars or something similar! A little bit of training concerning personal training which was conducted by a kid barely out of school who looked like he'd never even been in a gym before! I was asking him questions that he couldn't possibly answer, his only response being "Let me ask the fitness manager about that question" not too impressed so far you might say.

It was 8.00am Monday morning and I had just signed in for my very first shift after two weeks of extensive training, and within ten minutes a meeting was called in the manager's office- apparently a weekly event-where around twelve trainers were present, in fact any missing would be subject to disciplinary action so this must be some serious shit I'm thinking.

The fitness manager, a huge bull of a man clearly on steroids stood clutching his clip board and asked the first trainer how much money he would be making the company this week, the trainer said "Three thousand dollars this week" as he made a note of this the fitness manager replied "Make it four thousand ok" and by the tone of his voice he wasn't asking, rather demanding. After he fired the same question at the first three or four trainers it was very obvious whatever the trainer responded with it wasn't enough. There's a pattern to this bullshit I'm thinking, no matter what I say he'll demand another thousand dollars on top.

So it's finally my turn "Nigel, how much are you going to make for the company this week?" My response loud and clear without hesitation was "Err, probably nothing, it's my first day" everyone in the room burst into hysterical laughter, everyone that is apart from the two managers. The fitness manager frowned saying "See me in my office after please" I already knew this wasn't for me and stood up and said "Forget it, I may as well be a car salesman as be a trainer here" and promptly walked past the two open mouthed astonished managers and straight out the front doors never to return again, and even to this day I absolutely refuse to step foot in this gym!

I knew I could make it as a personal trainer on my own without the help of the corporate gyms, and this indeed proved to be the case, sure it`s a money making business, what isn't these days? But do they have to make it quite so obvious? I don't think so. Another thing I particularly didn't like was that they encouraged you to interrupt and tell members they are exercising wrong if you see them doing something incorrectly. Sounds fair enough but when the person you tell snaps back saying something like "I've been working out like this for 20 years! Don't tell me I'm training wrong, I know more than you!" It kind of gets old very quickly, and even though my approach was always friendly, it was obvious my interference wasn't welcome at all.

MY OWN PERSONAL TRAINING BUSINESS

So the big corporate gym scene wasn't for me. After I worked for this `Big name` gym a very short time I then found the perfect place to work, in a small independent gym. I went down to meet the guy who owned the gym I had seen advertised and was very impressed by both him and his gym. He hired me immediately. Now of course, with this being an independent gym, I just need to find my own clients.

Until I got recognized, and started getting clients I kept my other regular job which was a good idea as I still needed to supplement my income as to start with it wasn't easy getting my name out there. I tried delivering flyers to the local community which didn't achieve any success, and walking the streets in one hundred degree temperatures wasn't the most pleasant of experiences, but it had to be done, it was all part of letting people know I was a new trainer at their local gym. I built my own web site without any help from anyone, and considering I knew nothing about computers that was especially satisfying.

After a few months, my efforts started to pay off as slowly but surely clients started to come to me. One client turned into two, two turned into three, and so on and so on until I`d built up a sizeable clientele, finally enough clients that I could quit my other job as now I was making money like I never thought possible. It was one of the most satisfying feelings ever being able to quit my other job knowing I had now successfully started my own business.

To my frustration I couldn't find anywhere in the area that would allow me to carry on from my current level in Ju-Jitsu as they wouldn't recognize my organization and wanted me to start again from white belt, I wasn't about to spend another 10 years just to get back to the level I was already at! A case of politics really like "Our organization is better than yours" type of thing. Disappointing for sure, but this is the point where I started developing my own style of personal training incorporating self-defense and kickboxing into the sessions. I wanted to offer something different.

As a trainer here I felt I was more able to work on my own style rather than training like everyone else, and in a much friendlier, and certainly much less stressful atmosphere. I was making great money and also having a lot of fun, this really didn't seem like work.

So, what could be better? Well, certainly not having the drama that was about to happen. At least I thought this was the perfect place, but it wasn't to prove that way unfortunately.

IS THIS PLACE TOO GOOD TO BE TRUE? OF COURSE IT IS!

When something seems too good to be true… it usually is! Sadly, this was to be the case surrounding what I thought was the perfect place to work.

Here`s my account of a crazy time that was spread across a few months based around the gym I happened to be working at in Austin, Texas. This all happened between June and September 2008. I happen to be the only real witness to much of what really happened in which I saw what I thought was a normal man turn totally insane. Driven by a crazy and overwhelming desire to seek revenge and financially ruin his ex-wife, but it really backfired in a big way when it was he in fact who lost everything, including his freedom.

The gym owner Brian Smith always seemed to be a very nice and fun person to be around, very knowledgeable about the job and always ready to help anyway he could. Unfortunately there were a lot of things I didn't know about Brian and his past, not least of which was that he was actually crazy! I was certainly about to find this out though. While the gym 'Viking Fitness' seemed like a very nice place to work with a nice easy going relaxed atmosphere, it was anything but professional with two dogs constantly running around while clients and members were trying to work out, and also a parrot screeching its head off usually sat on the owners shoulder, who would be regularly cooking food in the back room where he was illegally living, the smell of steak coming through the vents isn't really what you want to be smelling while working out. One of my clients actually asked me for a menu one night as they were convinced it was a restaurant back there!

I had spent around 6 months really building up my business from nothing, plenty of advertising including walking the hot Texas streets with bags of flyers which wasn't exactly the nicest experience I've ever had battling the heat, and no one ever called anyway! But it had to be done, had to get my name out there for all the locals to see and know about. At first of course I had to do this in my spare time around working a regular job as I wasn't yet making anything to help supplement my income. One thing lead to another and my first client came then another and another, and so on until I'd built quite a sizeable cliental, certainly enough to enable me to quit my regular job.

Around the same time as my business was blooming I had just split up with my girlfriend who

I was living with at the time, she had decided to move out of state and I had no intentions of leaving with her, not after finally seeing my business taking off after all the hard work I had put in to reach this point. I had no desire to move and start all over again, so that was that and I was looking around at various apartments closer to the gym as I'd been making the 10 mile trip 3-4 four times a day depending on when I had clients and as I was convinced this gym really was the place for me to be and expected a long and happy time working there.

When I told Brian about my situation he told me his girlfriend Paula was looking for a roommate, she had a 5 bedroom house that was way too big for her and she was never there anyway as she was with him at the gym every night, the rent would be cheap and as it was so close to the gym, actually within walking distance he suggested I rent a room from her. Seemed like a great idea to me as I didn't have to worry about looking for a place to stay, I could move right in immediately with cheap rent and save on gas money too. All sounded perfect! Unfortunately it didn't quite turn out that way.

The gym was exactly what I'd been looking for, and certainly a world apart from the pressurized corporate gym scene. This place offered a very friendly and relaxed atmosphere with clients and members all enjoying everything on offer, there was purposely no really heavy weights in the gym so we didn't get the huge bodybuilder type, you know the types that like to scream and shout and throw the weights around making as much noise as possible, so without that type no one felt intimidated. It was basically a really nice and fun place to be. Apart from me there were only two other trainers so we had both local and out of area clients, plus of course the local community people who joined as members each having their own personal combination of numbers to access the gym when they wanted.

So, all in all a very highly satisfying place to be, but of course sadly like most things when something seems too good to be true, it usually is and this proved to be no exception.

A VISIT FROM THE LOCAL POLICE

Everything seemed perfectly normal until this unexpected moment. As I was preparing to meet a new client at 3pm I got to the gym around 2.40pm just to organize things as it's always good to create a good first impression to a new client, as I was doing this I was suddenly made aware of two dark shapes standing outside at the door. Two cops had suddenly appeared at the door, so I went over to let them in thinking maybe they might be looking for a trainer. That was my first thought anyway, after all nothing bad or out of the ordinary had ever happened to suggest this was the start of the craziest story I had ever been witness to that was about to unfold right before very own eyes.

They asked if I was Brian, I told them "No. I'm Nigel a trainer here but he`s in the back I'll go and get him for you". I didn't realize they had followed me into the back of the gym. Actually as I told him two cops were here asking for him they were stood right behind me. They told him to come out into the gym where I heard "Turn around and place your hands behind your back, you are under arrest" He pleaded his innocence telling them "This is crazy guys I`m innocent, it`s the ex-wife you should be arresting" He was being arrested for harassment of the ex-wife. No talking his way out of this, he was handcuffed and placed in the back of the car and driven away, just as my new client came in with a very puzzled look on her face asking "Who was that?" I said "Oh, just the gym owner" Great first impression I thought!

He spent one night in jail and was back the very next day claiming he had learned his lesson and would now forget about her and get on with his life. This claim lasted one day then he was back on the phone to the police wanting to know why his ex-wife hadn't been arrested yet. The next week or so he was either on the phone to the cops or the IRS claiming his ex-wife had withheld thousands of dollars from them and he had the documents to prove this. It was later revealed he had in fact falsified these documents himself along with $14,000 worth of forged checks that again he claimed the ex-wife had stolen and wrote them out forging his signature. Also, around this time he sent out several very rude and nasty emails to most of his clients, of course claiming the ex-wife had hacked into his email account and sent them, plus he placed several revealing photos of her on the internet. Now he was trying to get her in trouble with internet crime as well as anything else he could think up!

During this time Brian decided the gym needed a change and advertised it as a grand reopening, and as a new local sign company was getting ready to open he saw the chance to get new signs for the gym with discount for being their first customer, he was never one to miss a deal! The signs were installed outside and looked great, he also had vinyl signs made for the inside of the gym that would go around the top of all the walls, as the sign installer was booked up for the next few days Brian decided he would install them himself after drinking one Friday lunch time. As I was there at this time I tried to talk him out of it by telling him it's not as easy as you think to put these up, but he said it would be easy, so with my help and drinking several beers while he did it we started. It quickly became a nightmare! As soon as we had finished putting a sign up it was already peeling off and hanging down the wall! After around three hours we had completed our task. The next morning the signs were all over the floor, the ones that hadn't fallen were crooked and the whole thing looked terrible! I'm not sure if he actually paid the sign company or not as he claimed they were faulty, nothing to do with him drinking and not knowing how to do the job of course!

The next day while I was training a young girl Brian was rearranging things in the gym with the help of another trainer. He was drunk and staggering around cursing. The girl who I was training had never been in a gym before and looked very nervous especially when we heard 'Shit! My head" he had lifted part of a treadmill up to clean underneath it when it collapsed hitting him squarely on the head! After I finished training the girl her younger brother had come in to pick her up, Brian started telling him how wimpy he looked and needed building up, the kid looked like a nervous type to start with but when Brian stood by him waving a hammer saying "Hello I'm Brian the hammer" the kid actually pissed his pants! Needless to say I never saw either of them ever again.

THE ALLEGED BREAK IN

Saturday night, all seemed normal as we sat around the large TV In the living room watching movies, after a few hours Brian suddenly got up and left the house claiming he needed something urgently from the gym office. He returned 5 minutes later empty handed. I remember asking him if he got what he went over there for. He seemed unable to answer this and looked very uncomfortable then claimed he had forgotten what he actually went for! Around 11pm that night I went to the local store to get water, as I drove past the gym I noticed the gym office lit up and the office door wide open. I didn`t think anything strange just that Brian must have gone back over there. When I returned home to my surprise both Brian and Paula were still watching movies. I completely forgot to tell him the lights were still on over at the gym.

When I got to the gym early Monday morning Brian was acting really paranoid and panicking saying "Don't touch anything, the ex-wife has broken in last night and cops are coming" I asked him how he was so sure he knew she had broken in. He claimed only she had a key to the office door. When he told me he found the door open and office light on I started thinking back to late Saturday night when I had seen this. Strange thing was nothing had been stolen apart from a tax document which was later found in the back of the gym. Surely if someone was to break in they wouldn't have overlooked the lap top and the pile of blank checks in that office. I reminded him whoever broke in would be on the security camera, he quickly ran into the back then came back claiming it hadn't been turned on. I suspected he erased the entire recording from the weekend. None of this really sounded too convincing to me at all and was going to tell him to reconsider telling the cops any of this crazy sounding story.

Before I could say anything my next and newest client-Austin author Martha Flint had arrived-we had just started our session when the cops arrived. Brian gave them a statement, I was really surprised when I heard what he was saying, I'm no detective but I could see right through everything he was saying, so I could only imagine what the cops were thinking, and certainly by the look on the cops face taking the statement he saw through it too!

The first few days of this week Brian was regularly on the phone with the local police department really pushing that his ex-wife should be arrested for this alleged break in. First time I'd really heard him raise his voice as he shouted down the phone accusing the cops of not doing their job properly! Not the best way to handle the situation I was thinking, frustrated as obviously as the cops didn't believe anything he was saying at this stage. Everyone was advising him just to forget about his ex-wife and get on with his life and concentrate on the business, but this now was very quickly turning into a very unhealthy obsession and really was the only thing he wanted to talk about now.

The thing I remember about this day the most was the crazy wild look in his eyes as he trained his last client of the day, several other people noticed this too. You could almost feel something unusual was about to happen. He had also spent much of the day creating contracts for Paula, another trainer and myself that he fully expected us to sign that stated we would be responsible for paying the rent! In exchange we could keep all the money we made training our clients. As he was supplying all the equipment he would pay nothing! Something I would again hear later on. The deal we already had with him was every time we trained a client we would give him $10. We were more than happy with the current deal and certainly wouldn't consider this ridiculous contract he had made. As he was way behind on rent he was of course trying to pass on his considerable debt on to us! Nice try Brian, thanks but no thanks!

THE DAY BEFORE THE GUN SIEGE

On this particular Tuesday morning I was scheduled to train two early morning clients at 5 & 6am, but both had canceled due to some stomach virus that was going around at the time, so I decided not to go over to the gym as early as my next client wasn't until noon that day. I decided to take advantage of the free morning and catch up on some reading I had been doing. I was actually reading the third Harry Potter book, never did get to finish that one, which thinking about it now probably wasn't a bad thing!

At 8am my good friend and client Jane Brown called me saying she was unable to get into the gym and that all the electric was off and a notice had been placed in the window on a rough piece of cardboard stating in bold capitals GYM CLOSED UNTIL FURTHER NOTICE! I called Brian at the gym but no one answered, things starting to seem very strange at this point! More people were calling me now asking why the gym was closed. By this time we had Brian's girlfriend Paula and the local cat vet Dr. Roberts all trying to find a way in and see what had happened to Brian. After several more hours Brian finally answered the phone saying "We are closed now and out of business, see Paula she knows the details" and then hung up! Of course she had no idea what was happening like the rest of us.

Brian had scheduled a new class at 5pm from a local bank, he finally opened the door at 4pm claiming he had certain issues to deal with and would I take the bank class, so I agreed to do this on the understanding the gym would be open as normal the following day, as a trainer I operated my business out of his gym so needed it to be open. As I left the house and drove over to the gym I noticed quite a few cop cars around the area, in fact on every street from the house to the gym, when I drove up to the gym they were everywhere, I was quite convinced they would follow me into the gym itself, but didn't. Once inside I asked Brian what was going on with the cops everywhere. He said "They're coming for me, but I'm not going back to jail" then he quickly disappeared into the back room. He came back out briefly to remind me to sign the contract he had put together the previous day. I had already thrown that in the trash where it belonged! That would be the last time I saw him this day.

The bank class was difficult as ten showed up. Brian hadn't given them their fitness assessments as supposedly they were to come in individually during the previous week where he could do this plus tell them what to expect from the classes. This of course hadn't happened so I was faced with many that had never worked out before and with no idea what to expect. With a one hour notice I basically trained them as I would my own clients. And a big thank you to Dr. Roberts who happened to be in the gym at the time and helped out by keeping the class moving. After the bank class was over I went back home thinking maybe tomorrow won't be quite as smooth as we had hoped...and how right we were!

THE DAY OF THE GUN SIEGE

The big day itself...As I drove up to the gym at 4.30am I was relieved to see the place lit up, I punched in my code on the door and in I went, everything seemed normal until I went to the rest room, to the left where the living quarters were I noticed the hallway completely blocked by everything you could possibly imagine! Step ladders, boxes, tool boxes and yes there was actually a kitchen sink too! etc. etc. piled high right up to the ceiling.

My client arrived at 5am as scheduled, we started the training session and Brian appeared, and seemed very normal laughing and joking as he usually did, All seemed normal until he took his two dogs outside to do their business in the grass in front of the gym. When he returned he was like a different person walking from one window to another totally paranoid repeating they're coming for me, they're coming for me! He asked if I would take the school teachers class at 9am, so I agreed, he then said "I`ll be over at the other place, see you" what other place I thought? My client asked if he was on drugs as he seemed very strange, I said I didn`t think he was as I never saw any signs of drugs, just alcohol…plenty of it! Anyway that was to be the last I saw of Brian for quite a few weeks.

As 9am approached, the school teachers started slowly drifting in, we had around 8 in the class. Ten minutes later at 9.10am I noticed cops driving very fast past the gym and blocking off the road at both intersections outside the gym. As the police activity increased outside Dr. Roberts the cat vet came over and informed me Brian was in the back with several loaded guns threatening to commit suicide, and that Brian himself had called the cops and told them this! Dr. Roberts said that Paula was on the way over and he was going to talk to the cops and try to slow things down a little until she got there. Apparently when Dr. Roberts walked outside the gym he was greeted at gun point and walked across the road to the church car park where the police were camped out like a small army!

Paula came about five minutes later, in tears she left very soon after, a minute at the most. Not even his girlfriend can get him to open the door. No talking sense to Brian today! So, by now there are cops outside everywhere, crawling along the bushes by the road, standing behind a dumpster at the top of the parking lot, everywhere I looked I saw cops! Without trying to panic the class I'm teaching I carry on with the session, I see a cop making a gesture with his hand as if to say get out of there, my concern is do they actually know who Brian is? They might think it`s me! it`s not until I see one pointing a rifle at the gym that I start seriously thinking of leading everyone outside. Then they are getting closer to the gym and banging on the window shouting "Get out of there now" This time I do as they say.

As we all walked outside, there must have been twenty cops with machine guns stood right outside the gym, I remember saying "I`m only from a small town in England, I've only seen things like this on movies" seems like a strange thing to say now but then the adrenalin was pumping at that stage. We were all escorted to a vacant building around the corner from the gym in the same little strip mall. No one really told us anything but we started seeing lots of movement outside including the arrival of the SWAT team! Who proceeded to run past carrying all kinds of guns, hooks, battering rams etc. etc. by this stage a small armored car was driving around, helicopters flying overhead, even snipers on nearby roof tops and behind walls. It really looked like the setting for a Rambo movie or something, just needed Stallone to come running past and it would have been complete! I remember one of my local clients calling me saying "There`s a sniper on my roof" I said "Well, ask him if he wants coffee he might be there a while"

Hour after hour slowly went by and we were starting to realize this is going to be a very long day, many of the school teachers had summer and part time jobs so they started to call in knowing there was no way they'd be getting out of this area anytime soon. Where the police had put us was just around the corner from the gym so we couldn't see what was happening, but directly opposite were two girls stood outside their works place, I opened the door and asked if they could see what was happening, they told me they couldn't see anything but they offered us food and coffee. I quickly ran across the parking lot into their office, after eating I began making several trips relaying messages. This was almost getting exciting now! Until the cops saw me and put an end to my travelling by ordering me to stay put where they'd originally placed us. That's ok I thought at least I got to eat!

After around four hours of being stuck in this room without information, the cops came and collected our car keys and drove our vehicles around to where we were and directed us out of the area around the back of all the buildings in the strip mall. The only information we were told was when a cop very early on poked his head around the door and said "we believe there`s crazy man with guns in the gym" No shit! I would never have guessed that! Back at the house I turned on the TV hoping to get an update on the situation, but nothing at all so I decided to walk back over there and see what was happening, the cops had sealed the entire area off so there was no way to get back over there. Most of the neighborhood was out looking over their fences trying to see any developments. Strangest sight was a sniper laid down aiming his rifle at the gym while eating a pizza!

All throughout the afternoon the police were outside the gym on the loud speakers pleading with

Brian to come out and end this situation, what no one knew was Brian had taken a bottle of Tylenol with a bottle of ever clear quite a few hours before so had actually passed out long before the excitement really got going.

The afternoon passed and it was only just getting to make the news, the news crews were out in force by early evening. With no developments it was a very anxious time not knowing what was happening. My two good friends and clients Judy and Pat called me and asked would I like to go out for a few hours as by now the whole thing was very stressful, so they came and picked me up and we went out for a few drinks that evening. People were constantly calling me during the evening. We drove back to the house at 11pm where we found the roads open again with very little police around. Obviously the whole thing had come to an end now.

Brian had woken up around 10pm feeling very sick and walked out the back of the gym where he was arrested and taken to Hospital for treatment. He later claimed he knew nothing of what was happening outside the gym that day. So, that was the end of the 13 hour gun siege. He was only awake for around the first two hours of it then had passed out due to the pills and booze he had taken, very lucky he woke up at all.

THE DAY AFTER THE GUN SIEGE

After all the craziness of the previous day I knew there would be no way I'd be working this day so had cancelled all sessions the previous night. Out of habit I went to the gym anyway as usual, if nothing else I could workout, that was the idea anyway, but when I got there the landlord had in fact had the lock removed from the door overnight, so here I am locked outside the place I work with no way of getting in. Another trainer showed up and we sat outside reflecting on the situation.

As we sat outside the gym around 9am I was joined by one of Brian's regular clients and local resident James Johnson, we sat outside going over the events of the previous day both finding it hard to believe it had really happened. Many people stopped to ask us the latest news, but there really wasn't anything new to tell. We were later joined by Dr. Roberts who had arranged to meet the landlord to discuss the situation. Apparently the landlord had already decided to close the place permanently as he was tired of dealing with Brian.

After checking the damage in the back rooms the landlord was horrified at the state of the place. He was also evicting Brian due to the fact he was living in the back of the gym which was against the rules on the lease. The landlord told us he had his suspicions of this and said in his own words "When I saw the amount of dog shit outside I figured he was living here" Dr. Roberts got the landlord to change his mind and reopen the gym by very kindly offering to take full responsibility to keep it open. So at least we could carry on as normal and train our clients. Naturally, the reaction amongst my clients was one of total shock and horror that this friendly and funny guy who they saw on a daily basis was in fact crazy! In particular I remember my best kickboxing client and fellow `Brit` Angela Ingram being very disturbed by the fact that someone so crazy had access to these guns while she was working out late each night, when you consider Angela had only recently become a Mother for the first time her concern was well justified.

After a couple of days we went to visit Brian in hospital, there was a cop in the room at all times while he was in there, apparently this is regular procedure for this kind of situation. He was in surprisingly good shape considering the damage he could have sustained from the booze and pills he had swallowed. He claimed he knew nothing of what had happened and was very apologetic surrounding his actions and claimed business would be back to normal as soon as he was released, he also claimed he'd had enough of trying to get back at his ex-wife and was ready to let it go once and for all and channel his time and energy into something positive instead.

Brian was released from regular hospital then spent the next two weeks in a mental hospital, after which he moved into the house with Paula. Around another month passed of constant fighting between the two of them, if ever two people were never meant for each other it was Brian and Paula, like oil and water they simply do not mix together at all! Things were getting pretty crazy in the house by now and you could tell it was only a matter of time until something major happened. This particular weekend Brian was busy drawing up plans for the following week when he claimed he was to get his gym back, which of course wasn't true but he had managed to convince himself it was!

He had plans to take over the large grass area outside the gym and turn it into a dog training school! The dogs would be training outside while the owners were working out inside the gym. He showed me several detailed drawings of dogs working out with weights! By now of course I'm fully aware I'm dealing with someone who to put it kindly isn't all there! It was very hard not to laugh at those drawings! The landlord had made it quite clear in writing that under no circumstance would he allow Brian ever to return to gym as before.

So that left the matter of all the equipment still locked up in the gym, as far as I know Brian did in fact actually own all of that. Now he was busy finding a new location to open a new gym, when no one would offer him a new location he suddenly placed an ad on Craigslist selling all the gym equipment! Kind of difficult to sell something you don`t have access too. His next idea was to break in and retrieve all his equipment and put it in storage but as this would cost way too much the new plan was to store it all in Paula`s house! Now things were really getting crazy.

This time he got lucky as the owners of the old goodwill building which was opposite the gym offered him their building to open a new gym. As he had convinced himself he was getting his gym equipment back and starting a new business he was busy drawing up contracts whereby Paula would pay for everything, and because he was supplying all the equipment he would pay for nothing! Naturally she refused to sign this crazy deal. Now the atmosphere really heated up and was getting unbearable in the house. He accused her of not wanting to see him succeed in starting up another business, and actually blamed her for everything that had happened to him.

He was acting very strange this week, I remember seeing him sat outside the house smoking a cigarette, having never seen him smoke before I said "I never knew you smoked" he said "Oh I just started today" I thought that a little odd as he was fifty years old at the time! Also at this time he regularly claimed he was in the process of suing the Austin police department for wrongful arrest and harassment. Good luck on that one! Brian was now like a walking volcano about to erupt at any time. It was obvious something was going to happen soon, and it wasn't going to be very good at all.

YOU KEEP YOUR LAWN MOWER IN THE LIVING ROOM?

Noon this day would be the last time I ever saw Brian, he was already drinking heavily. Tequila at noon is pretty heavy drinking by anyone's standards! I knew I wouldn't be back until the following day as I was going to be at the gym quite a few hours this day then head on down to my girlfriends at night.

Later that night I set off back to the house, it was around 1.30am as I was approaching the house, all I could see were flashing lights from fire trucks, ambulances and of course cop cars. I parked the truck on the next street which was the closest I could get to the house where a cop very quickly stopped me and asked where I was going? I pointed and said "I live in that house" his reply was "Not anymore you don`t, some idiot just burned it down" My first thought was ok; I'd better go to Wal-Mart and get a new shirt! Another crazy thing to think, but again the adrenalin was pumping! It`s a strange feeling knowing all you have is the shirt on your back! And I guess this now means I`m officially homeless too. Great! Thanks a lot Brian!

As I got there I remember Paula giving a statement to the cops saying "He`s such a sweet man, he really wouldn't hurt anything" I`ll never forget the look on the cops face as he threw down his note pad and said "Look lady, see that house? your kids could have been in there tonight asleep, people don't just start fires for nothing, there's something seriously wrong here" The cop had started the statement by asking "Do you really keep the lawn mower in the living room?" One of the strangest things I've ever heard in my life! At that time of course I had no idea this was the cause of the fire.

After giving several statements to the police we were sat in the drive way when at 5am the Red Cross showed up and gave us three free nights at a local hotel plus a cash card with a value of $350 which was very nice of them. I did actually get to go to Wal Mart and get several new shirts! Staying in a hotel room with Paula and two dogs was hardly ideal but of course when you find yourself suddenly homeless it's better than the streets! When I got to the gym Saturday morning my 5am client Sandra asked me "So, how was your weekend?" After telling her all about it she immediately offered me a room at her house. I moved in Monday afternoon. So Thanks to the Red Cross and my client Sandra my short spell of being homeless never really happened.

Here`s a detailed account of what happened earlier that night of the fire. Early in the evening Brian had grabbed Paula`s cell phone and saw some male name he didn`t know then accused her of having an affair! This was a regular happening. The name in question happened to be Paula's big brother, very big brother in fact at 6`5" and weighing in at 280lb. Brian called him and left a very threatening, nasty and very graphic voice mail in which he threatened to beat Paula to a bloody pulp and to kill her, and if her brother had the balls to come over he would get the same treatment.

I heard the actual voice mail and it was very disturbing to listen to. Well, soon after her brother came over with two bouncers, Brian was waiting armed with a large butcher's knife. The bouncers were not needed as the brother was more than capable of dealing with a very drunk Brian. After disarming Brian with the help of a golf club the brother gave him a severe beating and left.

A short time later while nursing a broken nose and probably hurt pride more than anything else (after all this was the guy who prided himself on being such a great wrestler and regularly boasted about how no one could take him down) Brian was throwing Tequila around the house trying to start a fire. Paula had the good sense to realize one way or another he was going to start a fire this night and ran over to a neighbor's house where she called 911.

So the fire truck and police were on their way before the fire actually started. While Paula had ran over to the neighbor's house Brian had dragged the lawn mower into the living room, took the gas cap off and lit it, and in the process tearing his left bicep. The house was completely gutted downstairs with smoke damage upstairs. They found Brian passed out upstairs and was taken to hospital before of course going to jail.

Before, during and after giving her statement Paula was constantly asking the police how Brian was, they finally radioed to the hospital where a cop said "He`s ok apart from smoke inhalation, Oh and a busted nose, mouth and black eye" It was later reported in the newspaper he had been punched in the face five or six times and kicked in the groin! When the landlord heard about the fire he immediately closed down the gym, which remains closed to this day. He was one of the first to be interviewed on the local TV news and certainly used the opportunity to let everyone know exactly what he thought of Brian, and it wasn't a good report to say the least.

Paula even now tried to tell anyone and everyone who would listen how Brian was so loving and wonderful and that he wouldn't hurt a fly. Now with the evidence of a burned out house as a backdrop hardly surprising that no one took her seriously and she was fast running out of people willing to listen to her nonsense.

AN UNWANTED VISIT TO THE DISTRICT ATTORNEY`S OFFICE

I received a voicemail from someone named detective Peterson from the local district attorney's office Tuesday morning with a message to call him back regarding the case of Brian Smith, the last thing I wanted now was to be dragged any further into this mess, especially considering it was around 6 weeks ago now that everything happened and I had now moved on with my life and happily working at another gym, as far as I was concerned this whole matter was in the past where it belonged, but when I called the detective back at the district attorney's office it was very apparent they didn't view it quite the same way and asked me to come in to be interviewed about the whole situation, not really wanting to do it, but having no choice I agreed to go over there the next morning.

When I arrived at 10am the next morning two detectives sat there with note pad and pen at the ready and began to document my every word surrounding this case. Basically, I was needed just in case Paula decided to lie in court, if so, yours truly would be brought in and give evidence proving their guilt. I was seriously praying it wouldn't come to that. They asked me to give my honest opinion of Brian before all this drama started. I told them I found him to be a very nice, genuine and helpful person and still found it hard to believe what had happened. Then they asked me what I thought of the relationship between Brian and Paula, I was honest and told them they were like water and oil, just two people that weren't meant to be together no matter how much they wanted to as they simply couldn't see eye to eye on anything which resulted in constant fighting.

Detective Peterson said "Although he's still protesting his innocence at this late stage we typically find 9 out of 10 times they change their mind and admit everything at the last possible minute knowing by doing so they'll get a lighter sentence, only an idiot would do otherwise, and as there's so many charges against him it's not a question of if he will go to jail but rather a question of how long he`ll get, and basically that's up to Brian himself" the detective goes on to reassure me "Highly unlikely it'll go to trial and if it did you'll only be needed if Paula lies in court so I wouldn't worry too much about it happening ok? If she did lie she`d be committing perjury and she would put herself in so much trouble by doing so, again only an idiot would do that" after about an hour they thanked me for coming in and said I could now leave. I left not really sure how this was going to end up, just hoping I wouldn't be needed as I was more than happy to try and forget this whole farce and move on with my life.

THE DAY OF SENTENCING

Well, the deadline passed for Brian to admit he was guilty and with him still protesting his innocence this circus like show was heading to court. Brian still very much believed he was really innocent and actually decided to represent himself in court! With him doing so, it made the whole hearing so unbelievable that no one else was even needed to testify. Brian's version of what happened was that he was relaxing watching TV when a mysterious man suddenly came in the house at 10pm with a lawn mower and without saying a word proceeded to set it on fire and ran back out of the house. Totally crazy of course, but this is the story he has stood by ever since.

Not surprisingly no one believed him, least of all the judge. The charges against him included fabricating and tampering with physical evidence with intent to impair, aggravated assault with a deadly weapon and arson causing bodily injury/death. As the charges were read out in court the judge gave him an extra 6 months for failure to keep quiet during the trial. Brian was sentenced to ten years in prison.

Brian Smith still refused to accept or believe he was guilty right up to his first parole hearing some two years later. He was however released a few years later having served around half of his original sentence in prison. His whereabouts now seem something of a mystery, but it's believed he's now living out of state after being reunited with Paula once released from prison.

We can only hope wherever and whatever Brian Smith is now doing he can put all this behind him and start a new drama free life.

THE GYM IS CLOSED DOWN, NOW WHAT?

So, after all that drama now what? The gym was officially closed down and finished once and for all with no chance of being taken over. It seemed like no one really wanted to step in and operate a business out of that location. Interestingly enough, it's still vacant today, years after this incident happened.

Luckily, I had made enough money to see me through the next few weeks while I decided what to do. Having had a taste of running my own successful business I was in no hurry to return to working regular jobs. That would seriously be a last resort.

So, slight problem at present being many of my clients had paid for big packages and now I have nowhere to train them! Most were very understanding, and still in shock over what had happened, nevertheless I really needed to find another gym quickly before clients started asking for refunds. That would really hurt my pocket big time! Thankfully it didn't come to that.

A NEW GYM, BUSINESS AS USUAL

When another trainer told me about a similar gym a couple of miles away, I headed over there to meet the owners and see what it was like. This gym was owned by two ladies, and was well established, and had been in business for a number of years, and thankfully without any of the drama I had experienced from the previous place. Interestingly enough, both knew Brian Smith, the owner of the previous gym, and both had their own horror stories surrounding him.

As this place was only a couple of miles from the last gym, I quickly contacted my clients to tell them about it, and all agreed to transfer over. Many of which didn't even come to see the gym first, they just wanted to resume their training with me, very nice feeling to have such a loyal following. So I had found a new gym, and it was business as usual.

I still train clients here to this day offering personal training sessions covering anything from strength training, weight loss, kickboxing, and self-defense. Something for everyone you might say.

ENJOY WORKING OUT AND STAY SAFE!

This is the final part of my story, the part that has a serious message, a message that I want to get over to anyone who may be thinking of starting out lifting weights. I don't claim to know everything, but from my own experiences and mistakes I feel that I'm qualified to offer some serious advice.

The first three years or so I pretty much wasted by throwing myself head first into this without any serious thought behind what I was doing, it was very much trial and error, mainly error I must admit. All this pain and wasted time could have been avoided if I'd have thought to seek the help of a good trainer to start with.

But then again having said that, looking back now some twenty plus years ago I'm glad to have made these mistakes because it really makes me aware of how a client is feeling when first coming to me for help, and I`m very happy to guide them away from that kind of start I made. I know firsthand the `No-Pain-No-Gain` attitude can be a very dangerous guide to follow and certainly know what it feels like following this style of training.

So basically, if you come to me as a client you will be getting well over twenty years' experience and I will be more than happy to give you value for money and really help you to the best of my ability to help you bring the best out of yourself without over doing it, and to safely reach your fitness goals, but to first start you out on the correct path.

Well I hope you enjoyed reading my introduction story as much as I enjoyed telling it, I know a lot of it sounds amusing, but it also carries a very important message about safety and starting off in the correct manner.

THE DIARIES OF A PERSONAL TRAINER

One thing about being a personal trainer is very evident, people really do take you into their confidence, and really do tell you the funniest, strangest, and most personal things you could ever imagine, some of which you really don't want to know in the first place!

Being a personal trainer at times can feel like certain clients are using you as a cheap version of a counselor by telling you all their problems and personal issues. So one thing is for sure, you have to be a good listener to stay successful in this profession.

Generally speaking being a personal trainer is a very satisfying and rewarding job when it comes to helping people improve their fitness, after all, it's not just their performance in the gym you are helping, but rather their total lifestyle of being healthy. They feel better in everyday life, like less stressful at work, and many times at home too. So all in all, you are helping people feel better about themselves physically, and mentally too.

However, like all jobs personal training can have its ups and downs. With that thought in mind here's a collection of 65 short stories, actually some of the most memorable short true stories I have experienced in my time as a personal trainer.

All names have been changed to protect identities. Could cause embarrassment to the people concerned if I used their real names. Also the dates and locations have been omitted for similar reasons. So, if after all that, you still recognize yourself in these stories…Too bad! Enjoy!

1

The clown that launched my kickboxing career!

You might well be wondering why this story is included in this book as it's not exactly based around any experience in the gym. I didn't know at the time but this was actually the start to my kickboxing career, and apart from that, it's funny and short! That's three reasons it's included, and the perfect story to start this book off with, read on…

One of my earliest school memories-apart from the tedious day to day life of everyday boring education, that was strictly governed by teachers who thrived on intimidation and bullying tactics, most of whom I`m sure probably wouldn't even qualify for the position nowadays-was going to some kind of crappy circus pantomime show. I was around 7 or 8 years old at the time.

So, all the school kids are packed onto several buses and it's chaos as everyone is excited about being away from school for one day. The teachers have their work cut out today controlling this lot! We`re off for the day and heading over to a neighboring city to see some kind of circus show or whatever it was, no one really knows and no one really cares! It's a day off from school that's all we know, and that's good enough for us.

When we get there the show starts soon after, nothing too special really, a variety of singing (out of tune) and acting (don't give up your day jobs, please)! Also jugglers (who can't catch), magicians (who are anything but magic), and clowns (who look pure evil)! Etc. etc. basically crappy second rate performers who are very amateurish and haven't a chance at ever becoming anything close to professional, amazing how I can judge someone's potential at my early age don't you think? As if I know anything! But I know it's not very impressive, but hey! It's better than being at school that's for sure!

As the show is in full swing now, to my horror, not to mention worry, a clown seems to be looking at me like he's picking me out for something, and as I'm sat on the front row I'm expecting him to involve me in this ridiculous show at some stage. Please God! Don't let him pick me for this show, I'm thinking to myself. This is the first time I realize I have a dislike for clowns and very soon a love for kickboxing. Unknown to me at this time, my kickboxing career is about to be launched in a matter of seconds!

The clown is now walking around carrying two buckets of water constantly looking at me, he puts both buckets down and picks one of them back up and is now heading directly for me, and laughing like crazy as he launches the entire contents of the bucket all over me! Expecting to get soaked in water I'm sat there all curled up on my seat like a wimp, resembling some kind of frightened little mouse as little pieces of paper float all around me! Unknown to me the clown had switched the bucket of water for another one filled with harmless paper similar to confetti that you find at weddings, and now the spotlight is on me and I'm the laughing stock of the whole theater, not to mention the whole school! This idiot clown has made me look stupid and it's time for payback!

Now, around this time Bruce Lee movies were all the rage, and all the kids thought they were Kung-Fu experts (me included). So without thinking I quickly jumped out of my seat and launched a beautiful front kick straight into his clown balls! Bull's-eye! He goes down like he's been shot. For a few seconds there's total silence-no one can believe what I just did, least of all me-quickly to be replaced by even more hysterical laughter from the crowd than before! I'm now the star of the show and looking down on my defeated crippled clown enemy shouting "Let's hear you laugh now Mister clown you bastard!" no response from the clown though as he rolled around the stage clutching his privates.

As he was out for the count, I was stood over him like a referee in a boxing match shouting out 1-2-3 and so on, the loudest cheer was when I counted to 8 and I had won, with my arms held high I felt like Rocky! I was thinking of kicking him again when I felt a hand suddenly grip my ear, which was soon twisted to the point of feeling like it was being ripped off my head (yes, they could do this back then and get away with it, imagine that happening nowadays? I don't think so). Anyway, I was soon ejected from the theater by a less than impressed teacher and given a standing ovation by the whole theater! Well, all the kids anyway! Then escorted back on the bus and made to write out 500 lines, can't remember exactly what now, but some crap such as `I must not assault innocent people in the future` I also added `That doesn't include stupid guilty clowns` which got me in even more trouble.

After the show the teachers wanted me to personally apologize to the idiot clown, but he backed out of it claiming he was too shaken and refused to see me ever again. Oh well, another victory to me! For a few days afterwards, back at school I was the main talking point, and some kind of hero with the kids which didn't last too long, as it soon became old news.

The clown deserved it for making me look stupid! Ever since I've hated clowns and loved kickboxing, an interesting and very early start to my kickboxing career to say the least!

2

Anything you can lift I can too…Not!

It always amazes me how someone with very little experience can totally dismiss someone else's experience and strength thinking they can lift the same amount of weight as someone who has lots of experience, and happens to be twice their size, and especially when it's me they happen to be not taking seriously! But when they happen to personally know me and also know I've been a personal trainer for a number of years it makes it twice as bad, as it might have occurred to them that I might actually just know what I'm talking about! And maybe, just maybe they might realize I'm a little more advanced than what they are!

One such example was a guy I worked with named Roy. He was ex-army and full of himself, always telling me how he thought he could match me with the weights! The session was just meant to be an introduction into lifting weights, I told him I'd workout with him just so he can get a feel of weight training, but not to expect to lift the same weights as I'm lifting, after all, it's not a competition between the two of us. Sadly, he couldn't comprehend that little fact at all.

I was by no means the biggest and strongest in the gym, but that's fine, as I fully understood my limitations and was happy with my size and strength, I explained I didn't start off this big and strong, I was once his size with no experience and understand the importance of lifting safely and not trying to lift too much too soon, just got to give it time and progress steadily. I probably outweighed Roy by a good one hundred pounds and with no experience I knew he would have to start off very lightly, but Roy on the other hand had other ideas.

Everything we did he would try and left the same weight! As we started with a few machines it wasn't such a big deal as he simply couldn't move the stack at all. Ten out of ten for effort but as his face was going bright red under the strain nothing was happening. I would reduce the weight around 70% so he could do his set, easy enough on the machines for two people to work out together even if they are miles apart in experience and strength, after all, it's just a matter of removing a pin. Free weights are not quite as easy as you're constantly having to take the weights on and off the bar, which gets really old fast!

Even though it was very evident Roy was frustrated with himself, he was actually doing pretty well, with a lot less weight than myself of course which he couldn't quite get his head around. All was well until we used the smith machine for incline bench press, personally I warm up with 100lb which isn't too difficult for this particular exercise. I did my set then it was Roy's turn, I told him just give me a minute and I'll reduce the weight a little for him to start with.

I took some weights off and left 20lb on the bar. Before I could get in position to spot him he had already jumped on the bench and unhooked the bar off the rack and crash! The bar came straight down hitting him in the mouth! His arms had completely gone and had no strength left to work with this light weight.

I did manage to get a hand on the bar and stop it hitting him with full force, but even so it drew plenty of blood and gave him a nice fat lip in the process! He had no desire to carry on after that and went home immediately and never returned to the gym ever again. Afterwards he said "I guess I'm not as strong as you after all!" No shit! Whatever gave you that idea?

He must have been pretty embarrassed as he didn't show up at work for a few days after, when he returned to work he told everyone he was involved in a fight at the weekend and that's how he got the fat lip! I went along with that story as I knew how embarrassed he must have been about the whole session, I kept asking him to come back but he just didn't have the patience required to benefit from weight training, he claimed he was sore for a whole week after!

He also failed to inform me beforehand that he had some kind of metal plate fitted in his head after an injury he suffered while serving in the army, and he claimed when he got home this metal plate was pulsating in his head for hours! He also claimed it was so bad he thought he was going to die. Strange thing was though, he never went to the hospital or even called his doctor, surely if you think you're in that kind of danger you would do one or the other, or both? I'd like to think I would have anyway. Sounds a little too serious just to do nothing.

He said this `old war wound` had prevented him from working out as hard as he could or wanted to in the past, and that he is way stronger than the workout he did with me suggested. Sounds like he still can't accept his lack of strength and experience. Funny thing was, the session wasn't bad at all, when you consider his size and strength levels he did pretty well.

Looking back, I'm pretty sure this was just another example of someone trying to do way too much too soon without even trying to understand or accept their limitations.

3

What's that smell? Just my client farting…again!

A perfect example of someone with less than perfect manners-or indeed no manners at all-was a huge giant of a man from Poland named Tomas. He stood 6`5" and weighed in at 280lb. This guy was as strong as they come and actually looked like a power lifter, probably due to the fact his diet was non-existent, which he was fine with as his only goal was to get big and strong which he already was, he was a natural and achieved huge strength gains after only a few months of training.

The fact he was a truck driver certainly didn't help his diet as he must have put every piece of junk food in his mouth he could find on a daily basis! He claimed the training gave him a huge appetite, personally I believe he was just a compulsive eater.

Now it's one thing when a client makes it obvious they have no interest in eating a healthy diet, but why do they feel the need to fart in the gym without even trying to cover it up and stink the place out? And it made no difference who or how many were in the gym. Tomas would let rip whenever he felt the need, which seemed to be quite often, even when ladies were in there working out it made no difference to him! He was a nice enough guy with a friendly personality, but surely at his age of 45 years he should know better, just common decency you would think. But he had no shame at all it seemed.

He liked to finish every session with 10 minutes of sit ups, not because he wanted to reduce his expanding waste line, but rather he claimed it would help him get rid of excess gas, great! Just what we need! So we would place him as far away in the corner of the gym as possible. It would only take a few minutes before you could hear several people asking "What the hell is that smell?" as he worked out at 9am he had already eaten a heavy fried breakfast which was adding fuel to the fire...or farts in this case! And after the session he was ready to eat yet more junk!

This guy liked to lift very heavy, which is great but one slight problem being the heavier he went the more he farted! A good example being his ability to bench press 300lb for fun, then proceed to almost crap himself announcing "Ah, that's better!" better for him perhaps, but certainly not for anyone else as the stench clung to every square inch of the gym!

Being a truck driver meant he wasn't able to train every week which was probably to the relief of everyone else in there. The gym was actually more busy the weeks he wasn't there, with most people asking "When is Tomas coming back?" so they could actually schedule their own sessions around the times he wouldn't be there, not really good for business as no one wanted to be around him or even the hour after such was the smell in the gym after he had left.

The gym manager bought several strong air fresheners in anticipation of his next visit, as after a week on the road eating all kinds of junk food it was sure to be really bad. So, in walks Tomas who stopped dead in his tracks in the doorway looking around sniffing and saying in his strong Polish accent "What's that smell? The gym stinks like shit!" really? It didn't at that time but one hour later it certainly did!

Eventually the gym manager had no choice other than to ban Tomas as his antics were seriously hurting business. The last we heard about Tomas was several years later and it appears he had joined every gym in town only to get banned from every gym in town! Which lead him to buy his own set of weights and workout in the comfort and `smell` of his own garage.

4

Time to fire this rude client…twice!

Once in a while, you come across that kind of person who has the attitude from hell, the kind of person who will never be satisfied with anything you do for them, the kind of person who thinks they know better than yourself, even though they have no idea what they are talking about. The kind of person you have all probably experienced in whatever profession you happen to be doing, and the kind of person who is about to get fired!

I was actually warned about this awful person by her cousin who I already had been training for a number of years, who thankfully was nothing like this person, she asked me if I was sure I wanted to take her on as she was difficult to deal with, I thought well, just how bad can she really be? I was soon to find out just how bad she could be! I won't even bother to give this client a false name as she doesn't deserve one.

The very first session when I greeted her I got no response at all, I was trying to sound enthusiastic and said "OK, let's warm up first" she glared at me saying in a very bitter voice "I'm not cold!" not quite the start I was hoping for.

Everything I asked her to do she said "I don't want to do that" she would text me the day before telling me what we should do! For example, she would request we kick box the next session, so half way through this session she's complaining about kickboxing! Basically she wasn't happy with anything and thought she knew more about training than I did. I actually asked her if she knew better than me why waste her money paying someone when she knows best, that doesn't make sense to me, but that got no response at all.

One day she informed me she was having a large tattoo done the day before our next session, but she'd still come because she's tough, whatever! I tried to tell her there's no way she will feel like working out with a tattoo done less than 24 hours on her body, so why not cancel the next session now so she could relax that day. She said she knew her body better than I did and she could handle it, ok I thought, there's no talking sense to some people. Sure enough the morning of the next session she cancelled, not because of the tattoo or so she claimed, but rather she had too much to do that day! Don't you just love people who won't admit they were wrong? Her cousin actually told me she was in so much pain with the tattoo that she didn't even go to work that day.

Anyway, after several sessions that were truly terrible, with her being very rude, I thought enough was enough I sent her the following email.

"After thinking about that last session Friday, I am no longer willing to train you! Your attitude was awful and also noticed by everyone else in the gym. I`m tired of you constantly calling off at the last minute expecting me to re-schedule into an already very busy schedule. Most of all I'm tired of your attitude which seems to be getting worse with each session! I find you to be very rude and very unfriendly, the only time you speak is to complain. You have a constantly pissed off look on your face from start to finish. Obviously I'm not giving you what you think you need so I suggest you find another trainer, there`s plenty of us around these days, one that will put up with your poor attitude, because I no longer will. I don't need your money and I certainly don't need you. Good luck to you"

I sent this on Saturday morning, she texted me Monday night very politely asking when her next session was, this is the only time she had ever been polite so I knew exactly what she was doing, after I explained I had sent her an email stating I was no longer willing to train her, she claimed she knew nothing about my email, which was a lie because her cousin had already told me she had called her Saturday night complaining I'd fired her! So, I sent it her again saying "Now you're fired twice!" Thankfully, I never heard from her ever again, now there's a story with a really happy ending!

5

A fairy in the gym…No thanks!

People have many different reasons for wanting to get into shape, usually for their own health and fitness, but occasionally other reasons too, and this has to be the strangest request ever.

It was early one Saturday morning when I got a call from a guy named Rupert, who was obviously very distressed and obviously very gay! I remember the call as I've never heard anything like this before, this guy is crying on the phone! "Its Rupert, can you help me get my Geoffrey back?" I said "err, probably not, but I can train you" I honestly thought this was a friend playing a joke on me, until I realized this guy was for real and it wasn't a joke. He`s actually talking to me like I already know him, took a few seconds to realize I have no idea who this is and most likely don't want to know who this is either! The kind of person you get the creeps from!

He seemed to feel the need to tell me in great detail about how his boyfriend had dumped him for a younger man, so he thought if he gets in shape it will help him get this guy back. Oh, and he told me he already has a great body just needs toning up a little. I wasn't too convinced about him saying he already had a great body. Anyway after listening to this drama queen and his nonsense as long as I possibly could without hanging up on him, we arranged the first session, not one I can honestly say I was looking forward to! Just had a feeling this was going to be a total waste of time, and that's exactly what it proved to be.

The day of the first session was a total joke! This guy came prancing into the gym like a fairy! His gym outfit consisted of a white vest and pink shorts that looked a few sizes too small. He was stood there flexing these non-existent muscles saying "See, told you I had a great body" when in actual fact he had no muscle at all, painfully skinny man with a large beer gut! It was still really hard to believe this wasn't a joke and half expected a camera crew to walk in behind him with some crazy TV presenter announcing that I'm the latest victim of a practical joke, but there was no camera crew or crazy TV presenter, just this clown by himself! He had a very strong smell of mouth wash about him, God only knows what he'd just been doing before coming to the gym!

He then starts telling me he has a serious back, shoulder, ankle and knee injury that prevents any strenuous exercise, but still claims he can do anything in the gym and requests we work out very hard! I`m thinking what an idiot this man is. So we start off with a 5 minute warm up on the treadmill that he claims is going too fast! Not a great start considering he claimed he can do anything only a few minutes previously. He's almost in tears as he starts to tell me yet again of his boyfriend who left him.

He`s sounding like some kind of preacher spreading the word on what it's like to be gay! Each to his own, but this isn't what I want to be listening to at all. So, after the warm up I very quickly decide to destroy this guy with a few exercises just to see the back of him, hoping he will never come back ever again!

The session lasts just 25 minutes when he claims he has some unfinished business he had forgotten about! He can't get out the gym quick enough saying he`ll call to confirm his next session. I knew he never would, and he didn't…Thank God!

6

Ex-Army client who can do anything…Really?!

For the most part being a personal trainer, the clients I get are nice people and sensible and realize they are coming to me knowing I can give them something they know they cannot do by themselves, after all this is not a cheap service, so why pay a trainer big money if you can do it by yourself? That wouldn't make sense at all.

Now occasionally of course you get the big headed person who claims they know it all, but yet seriously know nothing about training, and prove this every time they open their mouths! I got an email from a guy named Paul, who claimed he was ready to start training again after a few months out of the gym, to say this guy was full of himself would be an understatement. This is the actual email he sent me….

"Hi, my name is Paul, I'm looking for a trainer and after seeing your web site you're the one I want to train me, let me know when we can start training please. I'm ex-army and can do anything you care to throw at me. I'm 6 feet tall and weigh 170lb muscular and very strong. I've served in Iraq and

Afghanistan several times as a sniper and can do everything from driving tanks to flying helicopters. I'm one of the fittest and strongest people you will have ever seen. Only an ankle injury prevented me from becoming a Navy Seal, if you're familiar with Navy Seal training you will have heard about `Hell Week` Well, while most people struggle badly with this, I found it very easy, and only a severely twisted ankle on the last day of this week prevented me from completing this. So, I need you to push me very hard to get me back in top shape again, it will be very easy for me, and I'll be your best ever client like a model client for others to try to follow that aren't as good as me"

Now there's nothing wrong with confidence, but there's also a big difference between confidence and arrogance. Flying helicopters? Driving tanks? Sniper? Very impressive indeed, but why do I need to know all this? After all, he's coming to me for personal training not as some kind of Rambo figure who is preparing to go on some secret mission to save the world! So, I wasn't sure what to expect from this guy, if his ability lives up to his arrogance then he will be an outstanding client for sure. For a small word "If" can be a very big word at times.

When Paul first walked into the gym he looked like he had never worked out in his life before, in fact, when I saw him it didn't even cross my mind that was him, I thought for sure he was another trainers client. We started off with a steady walk on the treadmill. He was already saying it was too easy for him! I mean, just how hard does a warm up need to be? This was the type of guy that wanted to lift too heavy, too fast with no thought to correct form or safety, basically he was doing everything wrong and he wasn't prepared to listen to anything I said. Also, all the time he's telling me these army stories which are becoming very boring indeed.

After only 15 minutes the session was over! He had to visit the rest room to throw up, he came out looking very sorry for himself claiming he must have ate something bad the night before. He had paid for 10 sessions, but never returned, I tried calling and emailing but he didn't want to know. He never returned any of my emails or calls.

So much for the ex-army guy that could do everything. Army? Maybe he meant the Salvation Army!

7

The drama queen and his dramatic panic attack!

You do meet a wide variety of people when doing this job, a real cross section of the general public for sure. From the fit to the unfit, from the serious to the not so serious, from the smart to the crazy etc. etc. the list of opposites is endless. Then of course there's always the good old drama queen, which I've found to be way worse when it happens to be a guy!

Brian came to me because a friend of his who I had been training for a number of years had recommended my services to him, this guy was a total wimp! Nice enough, but a total wimp for sure! He seemed to enjoy the type of session that would never see him get out of first gear, which is totally pointless and will never see any results, especially considering Brian was desperate to get fit and in particular see his growing beer gut disappear!

This was going to be a long road for Brian to travel down in order to achieve his goal, and taking into consideration his love of chain smoking, drinking beer and whiskey every night and on top of that a bad diet, I wasn't too convinced this was going to be very successful. He seemed to be doing reasonably well, but every time I tried to step up the training he would start panicking claiming he was scared of having a heart attack so every time we would drop it back down achieving nothing as usual.

One particular Saturday he claimed he was very rested and ready for a much more challenging workout, I thought yes! At last, now we can really make progress. How wrong I was. This was to be one of the strangest sessions I've ever experienced. We almost completed the full session when all of a sudden he started panicking and pacing around the gym like some kind of marathon runner on speed! I told him to sit down and practice his breathing like I'd taught him, in through the nose, out through the mouth to keep the heart rate down. He tried this for a few seconds then suddenly jumped up and then threw himself down and started to roll around the gym floor, he looked like a fish out of water at this stage. He was really playing the role of drama queen today, with the gym being his stage. The only audience today was me and another trainer who couldn't believe what he was seeing!

Little did I know Brian was only just warming up, just when I thought this can't get any more dramatic, he suddenly pulls off his shirt and is now flipping around the gym floor half naked! I manage to direct him into the lounge area where hopefully he will calm down. Imagine the scene, I'm sat there very calmly while this guy is going crazy on the floor. He suddenly grabs my ankle claiming it's a security feeling for him and will help, so I thought why not? If it calms him down that's fine.

He's not done yet though, now it's time for the show to really start. He reaches up and said "Hold my hand please" I can't believe what is happening now. He then comes out with a real classic "Hold my hand please, I'm not gay, I've had sex with over fifty women, I'm not gay honestly" He claims the doctors have told him it will help calm him down to feel the comfort of holding someone's hand, at this point I'm seriously thinking about knocking him out stone cold! That would calm him down for sure. So I'm sat there holding the hand of this guy who is panicking so much he's sweating more than he did during his workout. He manages to call his girlfriend to come and pick him up, who is new to the area and drives straight past the gym exit on the highway and is now totally lost. This freaks him out more than ever.

The phone calls between them get heated as both are now panicking, after around 30 minutes he's that exhausted he actually calms down enough to compose himself and get ready to walk out of the gym and down the road so he can be picked up. As he leaves I'm watching out of the window, he's walking down the road like a drunk staggering all over, I quickly lock the door and make my escape out of the back door where my truck is and drive off. I had visions of him coming back and treating us to a repeat performance of his one man panic show….No thank you! Once was enough.

The next session he apologies profusely about this incident claiming he had stayed up all night drinking, and had actually drank a whole bottle of whiskey the night before his session! Now considering his training session was at 9am, anyone who would drink a whole bottle of whiskey the night before their training session obviously isn't the slightest bit taking it seriously at all. Lack of priorities and all that, not to mention common sense.

He came for a few more sessions then quit, which I was ok about as he was a complete joke, but he did provide me with that unbelievable, and unforgettable experience.

8

Crazy excuses not to workout!

After a while doing this job you can soon tell who really wants to work out and who doesn't. The clients who truly understand they will only get back what they put into their training and the ones who don't even want to be there but come anyway expecting results without even trying.

Then of course you get the ones that pay but cancel almost every session, instead of being honest with themselves and me and just admitting it's not for them, they use the craziest excuses not to be there for their workouts, which I always find so strange, I mean, it's not like I made them sign up in the first place, it was their choice to come to me for help.

One such client was Sandra, a slightly overweight lady who came to me wanting to lose 20lb and basically just tone up, shouldn't be too difficult I thought. Unfortunately Sandra had no desire to put any kind of effort into her workouts what so ever. After three very poor sessions I received an email from Sandra saying she was sick and couldn't make it to the gym today.

As anyone can get sick from time to time I didn't think any more about this and waited for her next session. The day of the next session came around and so did another email stating now her husband was sick too, at this stage I'm not really thinking anything is too strange about this as people do get sick and pass it on to family members. At the weekend Sandra calls me to say everyone is fit and well again and she's ready and looking forward to hitting the gym again.

The day of the next session came around and so did another cancellation, this time the baby is sick, then it's the turn of the dog to be sick. OK, now things are looking a little strange, either that or this family has some very seriously bad luck with a sickness that only hits them on gym day! It`s very strange how that sickness only strikes down the clients who really don't enjoy working out. As the next session approaches, I'm thinking I wonder what excuse it will be today. I know she's running out of family members to get sick so this should be interesting. Sure enough the morning of the next session arrives along with the best excuse yet, her cat has just got food poisoning! Really? I don't think so.

So, in the space of two weeks Sandra got sick, her husband got sick, her baby got sick, her dog got sick and now her cat got sick, all on gym day of course, Whatever! Maybe next her goldfish will be the latest victim, some freak accident in its goldfish bowl perhaps!

By this time, I had already crossed her off my schedule long before she could come up with any more excuses. Needless to say, she never came back, and I never heard from her ever again either. Oh well, no big loss.

9

Why am I not losing weight?

One of the biggest and most common of problems is getting clients to stay on a healthy diet, after all, why waste money on a trainer if you're going to ruin the whole thing by eating junk food, doesn't make sense really.

A healthy diet and exercise really go together, like a perfect marriage if you only have one working it's not going to work, and will really slow down results, or stop any results altogether. Considering most people are looking for weight loss these days most clients will quit long before they see results because of their inability to follow a structured diet.

In the fast pace of modern day life everyone seems to be looking for a `quick fix` when it comes to exercise, but in reality there really aren't any magical pills or magical diets to get you that look you so desire. Just mainly having the discipline to work out regularly and eat correctly. It's not that difficult, calories in versus calories out! It's that simple, unless there's a thyroid issue of course, but generally speaking it's a lack of discipline that's to blame.

One such client was Joe, who obviously liked his food but yet wasn't too overweight. He came to me claiming to have tried every diet going but nothing would work for him. After training Joe for 3 months we were making great progress in the gym apart from of course his weight loss. His pant size had gone down a few sizes but not his weight. If anything his weight had increased a few pounds.

He claimed to be eating a good diet of salad, fruit & veg with no junk food at all or any alcohol, so this was a mystery as to why he wasn't losing weight…or was it? I had my suspicions about Joe`s diet so asked him to keep a food log for 2 weeks so I could see what exactly he was eating. When I studied this food log all seemed fine with oatmeal for breakfast, grilled chicken breast for lunch, Tuna salad for dinner with no snacking etc. on paper his diet looks perfect…if indeed it`s honest and accurate, which I highly doubted!

Now of course when a client gives you a food log, what they write down and what they are actually eating can be two very different things, this is what I suspected was the case with Joe, but of course I couldn't very well prove my suspicions. I gave him the benefit of the doubt, after all, why lie about it? He would only be hurting himself by doing so. He's the one that's paying me, I'm not paying him.

One morning I happened to be going into the local grocery store, when I saw a familiar figure coming out with a full basket of groceries, yes Joe! His basket consisted of several large bottles of soda, a couple bags of large potato chips, several packs of Guinness and many different boxes of cookies. Before I could say anything, a very red faced Joe said "Err, I'm shopping for my neighbor who's too sick to come shopping this week" I told him what a kind thought, I also gave him one of my business cards to pass on to his neighbor who must be in pretty bad shape to be eating this kind of crap!

Have you noticed when someone is lying to you, they seem to have an inability to look you in the eyes? Their body language gives them away every time as they try to convince you that the crap they're telling you is the truth. Whatever! Joe had been busted, and he knew it! He never did return to the gym either.

10

The generous stripper client!

It`s always a bonus to get a new client that's already in shape, and this was the case with Karla, who was quite open about her profession of being a stripper, claiming she was already in great shape and wanted to make sure she stayed that way. Understandable I thought, after all they make their living showing off their bodies and make good money so hiring a trainer is a good investment really.

When Karla came to the gym for her first session, I could see she wasn't joking about being in great shape. She really looked like the typical model. If she hadn't told me about her line of work I wouldn't have needed too many guesses to guess correctly what she did for a living, probably due to her oversized implants! This was going to be a welcome change to the usual over weight clients. Nice on the eyes that's for sure.

Karla was an instant star in the gym, not just because of her assets, but also the fact she could workout very hard with very little prompting, all in all the perfect client really. She had already pre-paid for 20 sessions, after the first session she opened her wallet which was packed full of bank notes and gave me a $40 bonus claiming my style of training was exactly what she was looking for to keep her body in good working order. The $40 bonus became a regular feature after each session, no complaints from me!

She had also told me to expect several of her work friends to contact me soon to start training too, and they did. So, we now have a gym full of strippers! Surprising how many male clients suddenly returned to the gym once word got around about these new clients, most interested in seeing the strippers than working out of course, but who cares? Business is business, and it's very good indeed.

All was going well until I received a call from Karla. She was calling from the local hospital. She told me she was hard at work the previous night when disaster struck in the form of a freak accident. She was swinging around the top of the pole when she lost her grip, slipped and came crashing down onto the stage breaking her right leg.

Unfortunately that was the last I heard from this generous client until a year later when she claimed she was ready to return, which she did but came back 50lb heavier looking like a totally different person. She went on to explain that after the accident she was too afraid to return to her previous job, so had spent the last year living off her now dwindling savings, her diet had also gone to shit! The training sessions were never the same as before and she quit training a few weeks later.

She had lost her motivation and her great body, and I had lost my generous stripper client, no more $40 bonuses for me!

11

Double vision or identical twins?

It`s always a good feeling, not to mention relief when you get hard working clients who are fun to train, and there's nothing worse than training someone who has no interest in being there. So when you get a good client with the correct attitude needed to succeed it just makes the time go faster and more enjoyable, this an example of one client who worked out very hard, you could say she worked out hard enough for two people! She also liked to have fun, and played an interesting practical joke on me.

I had been training Helen, a very attractive young lady for around 2 months with great results, during one session she told me her sister was impressed by her results, and that she was also wanting to start training with me, I thought great! Another client is always good news. She told me to expect a call from her sister Dawn later in the day.

Dawn called me later that night. She said however I was training Helen it was working great and she wanted to look the same as her sister. After talking to her we arranged her first session, one hour after her sister Helens next session. This wasn't requested that way to train them back to back, it was just the only available free time I had at that time of day.

So, after first training Helen she then left to be replaced by her sister, a few minutes later in walked Dawn, or was it? I was sure Helen had come back for some reason as she was dressed exactly as she had been during her session. I asked had she forgotten something, but to my amazement she told me she was here for her first training session.

She introduced herself as Dawn and said she was looking forward to training with me. I immediately thought this was a practical joke, but found it quite strange when she got her purse out and paid me for

20 sessions as Helen had only recently renewed, so why would she pay again so quickly? Taking the joke a little far I thought, but money is money and if Helen didn't mind paying so far in advance for her next package then I was fine with that too.

After two weeks the training was going great, but Helen was still carrying on with what I thought was this joke! She then asked if her and her sister could train together for one session as they were very competitive and wanted to see who had the edge. I was still convinced I had been training one person all along until the day of the double session. I was about to get a really big surprise though.

In they both walked, I thought I was seeing things, identical twins! Not only looking the same but dressed exactly the same too. Not sure which one had the edge as both had very similar ability, and apart from that I had no idea who was who. They were highly amused with my confusion and laughing all through the session constantly asking me who I thought each one was, I could tell they enjoyed doing this so I was pretty sure I wasn't the first person they had fooled this way. There was seriously nothing to tell them apart at all.

I carried on training them both separately for another 2 months, or at least I think it was both of them, but who knows for sure? They moved out of state soon after so no more training sessions, I miss training them as they worked out so hard, and were both fun girls too. This remains probably the most confusing situation I've come across so far as a personal trainer.

12

The cheap peacock that made my client quit!

When Ann first contacted me via email, her request was just to firm up a little, and lose 20lb. considering she had 4 kids and was only 21 years old she was in pretty good shape to start with. The way she attacked her workouts I had no doubt at all she would succeed. We soon got Ann in top shape thanks to her willingness to listen, workout hard and adjust her diet. She was pretty much the perfect client.

Strange thing was her husband would drive her to the gym, drop her off and go and get a large bag of food from McDonalds! He would spend the rest of the session sat in his car eating this crap! Not the best way to show support for his wife knowing she was trying to keep the weight off.

I remember when she first started her saying something about wanting a giant tattoo of a peacock done on her stomach in full color to hide stretch marks from her four kids. She was saving for that and it was going to be a reward for getting her stomach area flattened, makes sense to wait I thought, no point in doing this while you're trying to reduce the waist line.

When she had got the look she was after then she started looking around for a tattoo artist. The main thing in her search seemed to be the cost of having this done. I told her with this being a permanent thing it might not be too wise to be looking for a cheap alternative. Well, she soon found someone that was willing to do it cheaply and arranged to have it done at the weekend. As we figured she'd probably be a little sore after this we decided to cancel the sessions for the following week. This girl was pretty tough so she sat through the entire tattoo in one sitting.

She came to proudly show me her tattoo a few days later, it was certainly spectacular and very colorful, the art work was amazing, and it was looking as though her cheaper alternative had paid off after all, or had it? We had arranged for Ann to start her training again the next week, but the tattoo had become infected and Ann was now seriously ill with blood poisoning. She was out of action for 3 months during which time she had discovered she was expecting her fifth baby!

It was roughly a year later that she had recovered from the blood poisoning, and of course the birth of her fifth kid that she actually returned to the gym. Sadly Ann was now a good 40lb heavier than when I had last trained her, one week before having her tattoo. Now of course the tattoo looked terrible, the peacocks head had drooped so much it looked as though it was sadly hiding somewhere around her belly button. The whole tattoo was now very distorted and a huge mess, not to mention mistake. Sadly, Ann never regained her drive to workout as she done before and quit soon after.

I guess this really is the perfect example for anyone considering getting a tattoo, cheaper may not always be the best option as Ann found out to her cost, and I had lost a great client due to a cheap peacock!

13

I like working out so hard…for only one session?

This is without doubt one of the most memorable and funny stories I can remember. One particular client I had been training with great results informed me her friend Nancy would be contacting me, as she had referred my services to her. That's good, another client through word of mouth, can't beat that really.

She told me her friend was Vietnamese and was a very nice and funny lady but couldn't speak English too well, but she liked to use the `F` word a lot. Apparently Nancy was from Vietnam and had been over here around three years, her family owned a nail salon where she worked. That's original!

Later that day I received a call, and instantly knew who it was as it was a very excitable voice, and quite a funny phone call "Hello, this Nancy, I ready to fucking working out, I like to working out so fucking hard, me very fucking strong, you can do?" Trying not to laugh I told her yes we can workout hard, after setting up her first session she replied "Ok, fucking good man! Bye"

Obviously, Nancy appeared to be quite a character so I was looking forward to meeting her and training her too, just had a feeling she would be a fun client. I wasn't to be disappointed.

The day of her first session Nancy came around 20 minutes early claiming she wanted to warm up thoroughly so she could give it everything for the full hour, she was very eager to start training. She shook my hand with a very firm grip saying "I'm Nancy, fucking nice to meeting with you today, let's working out fucking hard yes" She proceeded to put herself through a warm up consisting of stretching that was more intense than most people's workouts! Nancy had arrived certainly looking the part in her very revealing looking tiny gym outfit.

The first session went very well, and it was very obvious that Nancy was very serious about her workouts, she was pouring with sweat from start to finish and never let the pace drop at any time. She was strong, fast, fit and very pretty, all in all, I knew I was going to enjoy training her for sure.

So, to her credit Nancy was as good as her word, many people claim to be very good before they start training with me but very few live up to their boasts, she did everything I asked of her and was a very high energy person for sure.

We completed the first session and Nancy left with her unique English vocabulary on display loud enough for everyone in the gym to hear "Fucking good working out, see you fucking next time" Everyone in the gym was laughing because it did sound funny, she wasn't trying to offend or be funny, it's just the way she naturally spoke.

The next morning, I called Nancy to see how she was feeling after her first session the day before, she said "Fucking good, I fucking strong yes" Well, I couldn't argue with that, I told her she might be feeling it the next morning, she said "No fucking problem, I can working out so fucking hard, me very fucking strong, easy for me" The morning of Nancy's next session I had a call from her, with her usual very excitable sounding voice, she said "Hello, This Nancy, I stuck on fucking toilet long time, cannot fucking walking, no fucking working out today sorry"

That was the last I ever heard from her. Nancy was very strong, no doubting that but I didn't think it would only be for one session. I guess the moral of this story is, be careful what you fucking ask for, as you might fucking get it!

14

What would I do if I get attacked?

During the kickboxing and self-defense sessions I have instructed over the years, one of the strangest and most common of things clients ask me time after time is what would they do if they were to get attacked?

Very hard to answer that one really, you either do one of three things you freeze, run or you fight back but it would be hoped you would do something but once the adrenalin kicks in there's no telling what's going to happen as it will be a spur of the moment action that you can't possibly predict in advance, and apart from that it's kind of difficult to tell someone else what they would do in that or any other situation. But as they're paying me they seem to think I should know the answer!

One such client was Rachael, who was outstanding at kickboxing and self-defense but every time I showed her a new move she was forever asking me "What would I do if I got attacked this way?" The only reply I could honestly give her was to say I honestly didn't know because people react differently, which of course is very true, and as I said before, once the adrenalin kicks in anything could happen.

Rachael was soon to find out exactly what she would do in this situation, one day while driving in a remote part of the Texas hill country, she noticed the gas gauge getting very low, as this was a very remote area and almost turning dark she didn't want to run the risk of running out of gas completely and being stranded in the middle of nowhere.

Luckily a few miles later she found a gas station, so decided to fill up there while there was still some daylight left as there's no telling how far away the next one might be. After pumping her gas she said she was struggling to get the gas cap back in place on her car when she heard footsteps behind her getting closer and closer.

She could see a figure of a man silently approaching her from behind through the car mirror, but as the mirror was dirty she couldn't clearly see who it was, or what he wanted as he didn't speak, but was still getting closer all the time. So close in fact, as the adrenalin kicked in, she panicked and quickly turned around unleashing a very ferocious front kick striking her attacker hard in the balls and laying him out cold.

Bull's-eye! Perfect kick! Just one slight problem though, this guy wasn't an attacker but actually the gas station attendant who having seen Rachael struggling with the gas cap was coming to offer his assistance, but very unwisely chose to remain silent as he did so.

Two lessons learned here, the good thing was at least Rachael found the answer to her question, she now knows for sure what she'd do if attacked she would fight back! The bad thing was, as for the poor gas station attendant, maybe next time he will say something before walking up behind someone taking them by surprise. Lesson learned the hard way, and painfully too!

I carried on training Rachael for a few months after this incident, we both laughed about it as she regularly relived the moment using the bags as the gas station attendant, and demonstrated her crippling front kick! She never asked again what she'd do if she ever got attacked, she found the answer that day!

15

The lonely lazy hung-over client!

Every so often you get the type of client who is just so lazy they are way beyond any kind of help, after all, I can only show someone what to do but I can't do it for them, many clients seem to think it's enough just to pay a trainer but don't realize they still have to do the work themselves, also quite often we get the type of client who sees you as their personal counselor instead of personal trainer. Mark was the best example of this.

Mark came to me very overweight needing help badly. so I figured this wasn't going to be easy by any means, many clients eat a reasonable diet but blow it with drinking at the weekends, Mark not only had a bad diet but drank three bottles of wine every night! But claimed he didn't have a drinking problem! Really? Mark didn't work as his family was very wealthy indeed. He even described himself as a very lazy person, none of this makes for a very healthy lifestyle at all, or a good client either!

We arranged the first session at 9am, Mark couldn't make it as he was still sleeping off the wine from the previous night's drinking session. I think we managed 3 sessions out of the 20 he had paid for, easy money for me of course, but not helping Mark at all. So I suggested moving the sessions to 11am, as that would give him two extra hours of much needed recovery time. He agreed to this thinking it was a good idea.

11am came around and Mark was there but way too hungover to do anything apart from a very slow warm up on the treadmill resulting in him pouring with sweat, I swear you could get high on the wine fumes coming off this guy. So after a couple of attempts he started calling off a few minutes before he should be there claiming this just isn't working for him. So I moved his time to 1pm, surely this new time would work?

Mark got to the gym no problem but by this time he was way too hungry to even consider any kind of exercise, his greeting every session would be "I'm hungry, buy you lunch?" Great deal for me of course as not only is Mark paying for training sessions that he's not using, but now also paying for me to eat lunch! This actually went on for a few years before I put him with another client at 4pm, this worked well for both of them, especially for Mark who got into pretty decent shape. Unfortunately this didn't last too long.

For Mark the training sessions were more about having someone to talk to rather than working out. He has since put on all his weight again and hasn't worked out in around two years now. He's a good friend but just has no desire to do anything apart from drink!

Oh well, I tried but this was a classic case of someone being too lazy to be helped, after all, you can only help someone who is first willing to help themselves.

16

Hit men in the gym? No, it's just my new clients!

Every so often you get to experience something really memorable, real fun characters that create an occasion you will never forget, one of those occasions you wish you could have got on video, this is one such occasion.

I had a call from a guy named Paul who had been training over at one of the big corporate gyms for a few months, when his trainer got out the hand pads one night he liked it, and wanted to try his hand at a little kick boxing. As that's my specialty he chose me to teach him after searching on the internet for a local kick boxing trainer.

So we arranged a date and time for a session. Paul asked me would it be ok if his friend Tony came along and a few other people also come with them, sure I thought why not? I'll put on a good show for them and keep everyone entertained. He said thanks and informed me that there would be a small entourage of followers with him. Interesting I thought, sounds different anyway.

On the night in question I didn't have anyone the previous hour so sat waiting in the lounge room by the back door. Suddenly the lights seemed to dim as in walked two of the biggest guys I've ever seen followed by a whole host of much smaller people, almost like two giant sumo wrestlers making their way to the ring with the whole crew behind them, only thing missing was the television camera crew and commentator!

The lights hadn't dimmed exactly but it was the sheer size of these two guys that blocked out the light! In they came looking very confident complete with dark shades and stood in the middle of the gym looking around, it must have looked a little intimidating to many of the other people in the gym as several were actually heading for the safety of the front doors leading out onto the street outside! Several people actually said later they thought a couple of hit men had wandered in looking for someone!

After we had finally stopped laughing at the `frightening` scene these two had just caused, and everyone had returned to the gym finally satisfied their lives were no longer in danger, I greeted them and showed them around the gym. When we walked into the boxing room Paul`s eyes lit up as soon as he saw all the equipment I had, not just hand pads but all kinds of punching and kicking bags, heavy bag and speed bag etc. and he really took to the kick boxing immediately and as soon as his remaining sessions had expired over at the other gym he transferred over to me and has been one of my best clients ever since actually losing over 100lb in the first two years we trained together.

Paul also persuaded his wife to start training with me too who has also become a regular client of mine. His friend Tony tried a few sessions but claimed a long term ankle injury prevented him from exercising and never really got into it and basically just came for support, and has since moved out of state.

Some you win and some you lose, but they both gave me an unforgettable experience that night that remains probably my most favorite moment so far as a personal trainer. Classic stuff!

17

Diets don't work! ...Especially when you've never even been on one!

You can very quickly realize who is going to take this seriously and who isn't, especially when it comes to weight loss as very few clients seem unable to accept any kind of responsibility and accountability where diet is concerned. This service isn't the same as paying for something at the store such as a television that gives you instant gratification, take it home plug it in and there you go! You have what you paid for.

This requires patience and time to see a change, including of course a diet! However, this particular client was definitely different as she made it very clear she wasn't going to even try a diet and wasn't concerned about losing weight in the slightest.

Margaret came to me 50lb over weight and quite content to stay that way, she wanted to kick box 3 times a week as more of a hobby than anything else, basically an excuse to get her out of the house for 3 hours every week. I wasn't quite prepared for what was in store….

Right from the first minute of the first session Margaret went into great detail about what she had eaten the night before, or more to the point what she hadn't eaten as she had consumed enough calories to keep an entire army marching for a week! This was all she talked about the full hour, fried this fried that! "You should try this and try that" she excitedly told me.

I tried explaining to her as a trainer I`m expected and indeed need to keep up a reasonable appearance, after all, who is going to hire an out of shape trainer? Her response "Your loss, you don't know what you're missing!" I`m thinking believe me I know exactly what I'm missing! By the end of the first session I'm feeling sick from listening to this non-stop barrage of junk food to the point I actually feel like I ate all that shit!

Apart from listening to this shit, she also tells me constantly how I'm preventing her from being at home sat on the sofa watching television eating junk! Isn't that the whole point of hiring me in the first place? I mean, she came to me, I didn't beg her to give up her precious sedentary lifestyle! And right now I'm kind of wishing that's exactly where she was!

The next few sessions are all the same, non-stop talking about fried food. Now she's telling me how she put on weight over the weekend and seems to be quite pleased with herself for doing so! "I can't understand it, my workout pants don't fit anymore, I've put on weight since training with you, told you diets don't work" she explains jokingly! I just laugh, but this isn't a good situation because if she starts telling people she's hired a trainer and gained weight that doesn't exactly give me a good name or reputation or credibility. So these kind of clients can be more trouble than they're worth.

She complains about severe heartburn throughout the next session and says she was unable to sleep last night and can't understand why, so I asked her "So what did you eat last night?" she amazes me with her response "Oh I had 19 large fried shrimp wrapped in bacon" then she goes on to explain she ate all that shit at 11pm then went straight to bed! That could have something to do with the fact you couldn't sleep! Just a slight possibility I think.

So Margaret trained with me for 4 months-before she quit to return to her precious lazy ways-and gained 20lb! That's a nice steady 5lb a month gain in weight! How wonderful! Her departing last words were "diets don't work" They certainly don't, when you don't even try to be on one! The only diet Margaret knows is the old see food diet, see food and eat it!

18

Midget throwing contest in the gym?!

Once in a while someone will invent some kind of new exercise craze that becomes very popular and takes the whole world over like some kind of plague! Usually something like a fast paced cardio workout, but on this occasion it just so happened to be midget throwing!?

"Surely not" I hear you saying, but I kid you not! I remember back in the day when midget throwing became an entertaining attraction, not exactly worldwide but in the local gym I happened to train at, every Tuesday evening at 8pm this packed gym-which will remain nameless of course-held its very own midget throwing contest where serious money would change hands. There were more gamblers in the gym than the local betting shop!

The gym was set up ready for this event in a back room that was a long narrow room almost like a mini runway, no planes taking off though in this instance just low flying midgets! It cost $5 to participate in this `sport` that would get you 3 throws almost like an Olympic event! No medals on offer here though just 6 pints of free beer over at the local pub for the winner, 3 for the runner up and 1 for third place, a little different from the gold, silver and bronze awards but looking at the participants I'm sure the beer held more value than any medals!

This ingenious event was created by the gym manager who also happened to own the local pub down the road. No shortage of participants eager to test their flying skills and at $5 it was too tempting not to take part, the whole event would take around two hours.

The willing midgets were put on a strict diet-as they could get heavy-and dressed in a flying suit, safety helmet and harness ready to be launched across the gym floor. You would get a run of 5ft in which to launch your midget, hopefully into first place. Typically the average midget would be launched around 5-6ft down the gym floor where a referee would be waiting with a tape measure almost like the long jump! Also a pile of mats would cushion the impact, no real injuries other than a few bruised midgets here and there! Until one fateful night that all changed....

So, enter `Tiny` a huge 6'7" 320 lb. ex wrestler and

bodybuilder who apart from being drunk on this particular occasion decided to try a different approach, instead of the normal long jump approach Tiny chose to launch his midget discuss style spinning around and around to the point of losing control-probably due to alcohol-and throwing the unsuspecting midget straight through the gym window! The midget was seriously injured and rushed to hospital and Tiny immediately disqualified!

Now this brought unwanted attention to this new sport in our gym in which it soon became illegal to do anymore. One really funny moment though was when the injured midget was interviewed from his hospital bed by the local news reporters, when asked if he thought he was actually helping to discriminate against midgets and turning this into a circus freak show, the injured midget looked straight into the camera and said "I'm 3'6" what the fuck else am I supposed to do where I get paid good money and given free beer!"

A few weeks later the injured midget lead a whole bus full of fellow midgets to protest outside the town hall carrying signs saying things like 'We want our jobs back' and 'It's hard to find work when you're under 4ft tall' nice try, but after that event it was banned and stayed banned, the injured midget went into a serious depression, gave up working out and drank himself to an early death! R.I.P. throwing midget!

19

Here`s my card, maybe I can help you win the next fight?

As many trainers at the gym didn't like to take on late night clients and finish work too late at night, quite often I'd be the last trainer to leave the gym and regularly locked up at 10pm after my last client of the evening. I never minded working that late so usually had a 9-10pm client most weekdays.

At that time of night it's usually very quiet but anyone could be on the streets, and considering at this particular time quite a few new bars had opened close by so now many more people were out in this area drinking, and with there being a dive of a bar opposite the gym quite often all the local deadbeats and undesirables were out and about too! Sometimes looking for trouble, fueled by too much alcohol of course. I was always expecting to see a fight any night, particularly outside that bar and one night I did.

On this particular hot summer's night as I'm locking the gym up, I hear a commotion as around 10 drunks suddenly pile out of this bar and start a mass brawl in the parking lot! From what I could see initially they either had no idea how to fight, or the booze has impaired their vision drastically as I could see very few punches connecting! Just heads down and wild swinging, hoping for the best.

Not much of a fight but it's very entertaining, so I sit in my truck and watch the spectacle unfold before my eyes. Eventually one group got the upper hand and seemingly satisfied with their `hard fought `victory they quickly take off before the cops arrive leaving their defeated enemies scattered around the ground looking and feeling very sorry for themselves.

Now, never the one to miss out on a possible opportunity to get new clients I quickly grabbed a hand full of my kickboxing business cards and walked over to the defeated and dejected looking losers of this drama, I quickly handed out my cards, and the ones still semi-conscious I leave one on their lifeless looking bodies telling them "Maybe next time you can kick their asses if you come and train with me, I'll teach you how to fight!" all I can hear are moans and groans and feeble cries of `Go away! We`ve had enough, please no more!"

Guess they must be delirious passing this opportunity up! Well, there's just no helping some people I guess, just trying to serve the community in and out of the gym! As I drive away laughing my ass off I pass several cop cars heading to the scene of the fight. Timing is everything, a few seconds earlier the cops might have thought I'd beat this motley looking crew up!

For a few weeks after this incident, there was always a cop car in the parking lot around the time the bar closed, no more disturbances to report though, and none of them ever did contact me! Oh well, perhaps they didn't fancy their chances in a re-match after all!

20

The trainer who wanted a TV...This bad, really?

With hard times quite often come bad and desperate decisions, this is one such occasion. Not a bad person but just someone going through a hard time and resorting to theft without covering his tracks....don't give up your day job!

As I usually have an early client most mornings I'm usually the first trainer to unlock the gym very early in the morning around 4.30am, I've done this so often I have my own little instinctive routine, after I open the doors I first turn on the lights, fans, and turn on the radio and then the TV. Slight problem this particular morning though, the TV isn't there! Weird as I locked the place up less than 6 hours ago the previous night and know for a fact it was there then. Something doesn't quite add up here I'm thinking!

The gym manager arrives a few minutes later who quickly checks the video of the security camera in the gym, and we see quite clearly a hooded figure sneaking into the gym at 11.30pm the previous night and making off with the gym TV, as this was a new 50" flat screen TV the gym manager calls the cops and explains what happened. To our amazement within 10 minutes three cop cars pull up at high speed, flashing lights and sirens blazing for all to see and hear! Impressive response but considering this crime took place 5 hours ago slight overkill we think!

When the cops ask to view the video we look properly at the evidence for the first time in any detail and quickly realize who this thief is, none other than a trainer at the gym itself! This particular trainer had a very distinctive attire that would set him aside from others in a crowd, and yes you guessed it! He stole the TV wearing the exact same clothes! Not the brightest start to his life of crime really.

The trainer in question was due in the following morning to train his next client, when he came in he looked a little nervous to say the least especially when we told him someone stole the TV the day before! He really went overboard claiming he was out of town visiting family the last few days totally unaware that we knew exactly where he was... In the gym stealing the TV! This was backed up by one of my clients who actually saw him shopping in a local store the previous night dressed in exactly the same clothes, this is how my client recognized him even though he didn't know him personally to speak to, but had seen him in the gym many times.

The gym manager happened to say aloud "Maybe we'll get lucky and the TV will be returned before we press charges, the cops are ready to but it's a pity to see someone's life and reputation destroyed over a TV, and they'll find it very hard to find a job once its revealed who they are" of course all within ear shot of this trainer/thief! The trainer remains in the gym for the next couple of hours really emphasizing the fact he was out of town to anyone willing to listen, by this time he's really sounding very unconvincing indeed.

The next morning I unlocked the gym as usual at 4am, as I stepped into the gym I went flying over something that was obstructing the doorway...the stolen TV! It was back, no guesses for who brought the stolen goods back of course! That was the last time anyone ever saw this particular trainer, guess he quickly figured out his cover had been blown and was too ashamed to return to the gym.

The moral of this story could be if you're going to steal something and be in full view of a security camera don't wear the same exact clothes as everyone sees you in every day! Or of course, don't steal in the first place would be even better advice!

21

If you lost weight you'd get better tips!

Sometimes it's better to think before you speak, but not always possible as it doesn't work quite that easy at times, the old brain isn't as fast as the tongue! I'm sure you've all experienced an occasion you've said something and instantly wish you hadn't right? But too late, the damage has been done and can't be reversed! Here's my own personal experience of this unfortunate occurrence.

One morning at my favorite breakfast place the over-weight waitress is asking me about personal training, I don't mind answering a few questions here and there but when you know they have no intentions of actually coming to the gym it gets a little old "I need to get in shape and get fit" she says for the twentieth time this month! Then starts complaining about how tight people are leaving small tips.

While she's approaching with a refill of my coffee my tongue suddenly over-powers my brain and blurts out "You know if you lost weight you'd get better tips" my brain suddenly kicks in leaving me thinking shit! Why did I just say that?

For a few uncomfortable seconds there's almost like a stand off! Both our eyes firmly fixed on one another waiting for that first sign of weakness, waiting for that first move just like two cowboys waiting for the other to draw his gun first! Am I going to apologize before she pours coffee all over me? What's going to happen? The tension is building! Like the end of a soap opera that keeps you in suspense till the next episode. Neither of us is giving an inch! Who's going to be the first to back down? Who is going to be the first to crack under pressure? Ok, so that's a bit over the top, but you get the picture right?

To my amazement she says "I do believe you're right sir, here the coffee is on me today" Wow! A lucky escape or what? Laughing to myself I think the coffee is better on you than me after being convinced she was going to pour it in my lap or something!

The funny thing was after this I would get free coffee every time I went to this joint! Which back then was pretty much on a daily basis! The waitress claimed she was going to start training with me but never did, but I was happy enough getting my free coffee, guess she thought my comment was really trying to help her! She remained fat and I got free coffee for 3 months till one day I noticed she wasn't there, when I asked where she was another over-weight waitress told me she had quit the previous day, oh well, guess that's the end to my free coffee!

The new over-weight waitress said "I hear you're a trainer, I really need to lose weight" I'm thinking shit! This sounds familiar here we go again! But this time I keep my comments to myself and politely nod my head in agreement and carry on eating before I say something that could get me in trouble! Not sure I could get away with that twice!

22

It's not over till the fat lady sings…or farts!

Advertising for local business can be hard, like walking the streets going door to door handing out flyers is time consuming, and not too pleasant in the heat either. But you can also make it fun too if you happen to have plenty of business cards with you, and if you don't mind being turned down repeatedly then you're all set!

As one of my favorite pastimes is always being on the hunt for new clients, wherever I may be there's always potential new clients to be found so I always have a pocket full of my business cards so I'm ready for such an opportunity to arise. Like a great hunter after his prey timing is everything, one false move and my target could escape-It's my personal challenge and goal to see everyone in my local town have one of my business cards whether or not they want one-This particular instance I was wishing they had gotten away.

I quite often find my victims in the local store, the object is for me to get one of my business cards into their basket without them knowing, occasionally someone will call complaining about my cards ending up in their shopping baskets! As my targets are over-weight people they don't always appreciate my gesture saying "Are you trying to be funny because I'm fat?!" thinking quickly I tell them "I paid a bunch of kids to hand out my cards and didn't know they did this, but it won't happen again sorry!" That usually defuses the situation and I then plan my next trip to the store.

So the scene is set in the local store, I'm on the hunt again following my latest victim around the various isles. More often than not the chase ends around the soda and chip isle! The object of this chase is to try and throw my business card into their basket without being noticed. I'm in hot pursuit of a very large lady who is singing rather badly all the way around the store. Almost like some kind of over-weight tropical out of tune Parrott!

On this occasion my victim is proving to be very elusive indeed and a real challenge! The chase lasts 20 minutes before I get the chance to walk past unnoticed with my business card. I finally get my victim cornered on the soda isle where she`s busy getting as many soda bottles into her basket as possible, I'm thinking is she going to drink all this shit herself as I make my final approach and get within 5ft where satisfied she thinks no one is around she lifts her leg up and lets rip with the loudest most disgusting smelling fart you've ever experienced! All the time still singing! I quickly spin around and make my exit heading out of the store as fast as possible!

Like all great hunters this is a case of the one that got away, defeated I have lost the battle but not the war! I'll be back armed with more cards and possibly a gas mask too! Like the saying goes "It's not over till the fat lady sings" but when she farts too… forget it! It's over!

23

You'd better get results…or else!

It always amazes me how clients have many different reasons for hiring a personal trainer, but even more amazing is how many of their partners don't understand why they can't do it themselves and save some money! Many really do resent them spending money on this, but like I tell them it's not cheap but at what price is your health? And besides that it's cheaper to look after your body now than to have to pay a fortune in medical treatment in later life when your health suffers due to lack of exercise. Most get it but still doesn't make things easy when their partners don't get it, and unfortunately they're usually the ones paying!

One such client was Abby, a young attractive girl who claimed she needed to lose around 10lb, no more than that really so shouldn't be too difficult but was under intense pressure from her boyfriend to get results fast and as cheaply as possible! When Abby first contacted me her first question was if I could charge her less than my standard rate, I said no simply because if you allow them to, many people will devalue your service and after all this is a business, perhaps she would like to work at a reduced rate in her job? Not likely and neither would I.

So, that little issue out of the way we got down to business, she explains her boyfriend is crazy and has actually threatened her with a beating if she doesn't lose the weight fast enough! After each session he was going to personally weigh her to monitor her weight loss! She said her weight has been up and down for a few years now.

This girl was terrified of failing and because of this the pressure she was under from both her crazy boyfriend and indeed herself was immense. I explained it's more about the diet than training to lose weight in hope she could pass this information on to her boyfriend, she did and his response was that of "Well he would say that, he wants to drag this out for the money!" with that kind of attitude it becomes pointless. Abby told me he had said "If you waste my money you'll be very sorry" no pressure of course! Maybe after he beats her he`ll come for me too? From what I've heard of this idiot a good beating would do him some good!

Anyway Abby lost 10lb in one month and quit under her boyfriend's orders! On the last session she confided in me that basically she had been starving herself to lose the weight quickly, I tried explaining that's a very short term solution and very unhealthy and unless you plan never to eat properly or workout again the weight is sure to return. She claimed she understood that and would deal with it when it happened, but for now her boyfriend is happy with her and that's all that matters!

Wonder how happy he`ll be when the weight returns? Thankfully I never did find out as Abby never came back to the gym, either he accepted the weight or maybe she got rid of him. Hard to imagine either those two options being true really.

So many controlling people around these days especially related to the gym such as this story that I get to experience first-hand, my question is why the hell would you want to be with someone like this in the first place? A simple enough question that people being controlled have no answer to other than to say "But he loves me" Yeah, Whatever!

24

Unrealistic expectations from a client's know-it-all husband!

One thing you have to deal with as a personal trainer are the many annoying clients who think they know more than you! Now of course if this were true I'd be paying them instead of them paying me, so get real people, you're coming to a trainer for advice, motivation and knowledge on something you don't know how to do by yourself.

I think that's a fair reflection on the situation but still many believe they know best, funny thing is they could save themselves some serious money if this were actually true. Would they like me to show up at their job and claim I know better than them, even though I don't know what their job entails? No, of course they wouldn't. So why do it to your trainer? Doesn't make sense.

This is a classic case of clients thinking they know better than me. I had been training Paul and Sarah for a few years, both very nice people but Paul was a know-it-all claiming such shit like it`s ok to drink beer and eat unhealthy and still lose weight as long as you work out regularly! Nice thought, but just doesn't work like that.

Working out will help of course but there has to be a controlled diet in place too. When a client really believes this nonsense you know it's only a matter of time before they start to question your training as being the reason they're not losing weight. Very annoying listening to this shit from someone who has no idea what the hell they're talking about.

Paul and Sarah had been coming to me for training on and off for the last 5 years, they'd come for 3 months then get the look they wanted and quit claiming they knew enough to do it by themselves, Good luck on that one! And of course within 3 months their weight had returned and back they come again, like constantly taking one step forward and three back! Nothing achieving this way for sure but they know best of course.

On their latest comeback, they have now made more comebacks than Rocky Balboa, they announce Sarah is pregnant. The thought of being a dad for the first time is very stressful for Paul and he quickly quits leaving Sarah to use the remaining sessions by herself which is fine with me.

Now of course, there's nothing wrong with working out while being pregnant, it's actually a good thing but obviously the sessions have to be modified somewhat and extra care is to be taken while working out, nothing too strenuous basically. Sarah's Doctor is delighted with her progress during the first 3 months of pregnancy and tells her whatever she's doing in the gym to keep it up as its working extremely well! All seems well and everyone is happy all except Sarah`s husband who thinks she shouldn't be putting on weight around her hips and thighs, sounds like a case of having a trophy wife and he's worried she will lose her tight body, never mind the fact she's 3 months pregnant! His unrealistic concerns carry on for another 2 months.

It`s now 5 months and Sarah is starting to really show the signs of being pregnant and next session Sarah has all these requests from her husband, her ass is getting too big, her thighs are getting bigger and her stomach is too big! Maybe Paul doesn't realize this is what happens when you're 5 months pregnant! Funny thing is Sarah tells me it's now 5 months since Paul worked out and he's the one that's really piling on the weight! Maybe he should be more concerned about his own appearance than someone who is 5 months pregnant!

When the time comes they have a healthy baby boy which they bring to show me in the gym, I'm shocked to see Paul 40lb heavier than he was 9 months ago but he claims he's got the situation under control and knows exactly how to get back in shape without my help, I highly doubt that but of course he knows best!

I haven't heard from either of them for a few months now, but they'll be back heavier than ever, that you can count on!

25

The client with no confidence!

Quite often as a personal trainer you deal with people with no confidence, and quite often it's usually due to them being overweight. The hardest step for them is actually having the courage to first walk into a gym, once inside hopefully their mind set changes, and as they look around they'll realize gyms aren't just full of super fit looking people or bodybuilders, but rather people like themselves, just regular people of all shapes and sizes wanting to improve their fitness and health.

No matter how fit and expert looking someone might appear to be, they didn't start off that way, everyone has had to start somewhere and usually the first step is to contact a personal trainer for proper guidance, I had an email from a potential new client that was different to say the least. This is the exact email

"Hi, my name is Eric, and I'm a fat piece of shit!" that was it! Short and sweet. So, apart from being overweight this also tells me Eric has no confidence at all. After a few emails we arrange a time for Eric to visit the gym and see what he thinks about starting a training program. I purposely arrange a time when I know very few people will be in the gym. Got to try and get people relaxed right from the start, make them feel welcome and hopefully they will think of the gym as being their second home.

To my surprise when Eric first walked in the gym I was thinking he must be another trainer's client as he wasn't what I'd envisaged at all. Not out of shape at all really, perhaps 10lb overweight but not really a big deal, and certainly not worthy of his `fat piece of shit` introduction in that first email I received. He looked very nervous for sure which confirmed what I had already suspected, Eric was suffering from major lack of confidence and not suffering from being overweight.

He went on to explain that his wife had requested he seek the help of a trainer claiming she wasn't impressed by his lack of exercise and energy, and he was a little worried he might lose her if he didn't change his ways, so here he is ready to take the plunge forward into a whole new lifestyle.

Eric quickly took a liking to the gym and my style of training which saw him shed 20lb in 4 months, with a sensible diet in place too of course. He stepped the training up to five times weekly and it quickly became a new way of life. Also he developed some much needed confidence.

Everyone happy it would appear, apart from his wife that is who later divorced him for spending too much time and money in the gym! As I remember it was her idea he do this in the first place. To his credit Eric is still one of my regular clients and has gone from strength to strength with no intentions of giving up!

A real success story for sure, pity about the wife though! Oh well, you can't please everyone I guess.

26

A professional fighter is coming…Or is he?

In most jobs you meet and work with people who aren't quite what they seem, you know the type, the ones who claim to be something they aren't, and personal training is no different. Dealing with people with over inflated egos is part of the job and occasionally you get the one that is very extreme.

The best example of this in my experience was when a guy named Richard called me claiming to be a professional fighter wanting me to train him just for one session, considering he lived around 200 miles away I thought this a little odd to say the least, why travel that distance to train with a total stranger for only one hour? Doesn't really make sense. However, he went on to explain that he would be in the area on business that particular weekend.

Ok, now it makes more sense. Just when I'm beginning to think this guy is genuine he said he was impressed by my reputation in the kickboxing world! Now, this is kind of strange considering I'm not a professional fighter and don't even have a reputation to speak of, I'm just the friendly neighborhood trainer, and nothing more really. This is the time I start to seriously doubt this guy's credibility. Something is strange for sure.

Anyway, Richard was persistent about doing this so we set up a time the following Sunday. He built his reputation up to the max telling me how one day he will be champion! And he's done this and he's done that. He reeled off a whole list of fighters he claimed to have beaten but certainly no one I had ever heard of before though. Even so, I told several of my kickboxing clients all of whom really wanted to be there to witness this professional fighter in action.

I asked Richard if he would mind a few onlookers during the session, he said he was fine with that and actually said he'd put on a great show for them. So the scene is set and we`re looking forward to this, after all its not every day we get a professional fighter in our gym, not to mention a possible future champion!

With 3 days to go I get a text from Richard claiming he's pulled a muscle and not sure if he'll be able to do his training session as planned, at this stage I can't make up my mind about this guy as to whether or not he's genuine or not, so I tell him no problem, as he's in the area maybe he could come and look around the gym anyway, even if he can't workout this time it could be good for him to see the gym for next time when he's in the area again.

Strangely enough, he doesn't respond to this text. The day before our session he texts again confirming he won't be coming as he has a family emergency and needs to return home quickly. Can't really say I'm surprised as too many things didn't add up. Out of interest just to know more about this guy I find his profile on Facebook, I match it up with his phone number as of course there's always more than one person with the same name, to my shock and horror this is what my detective work reveals…

Richard isn't a professional fighter at all! No big surprise there really. He happens to be a 55 year old transvestite cabaret performer whose stage show includes him dressed in little pink boxer's shorts and pink gloves! And to top it all this guy wasn't even in this area this particular weekend! What a total joke! Better be careful what you put on Facebook as it can make a liar of you! He doesn't even look like he works out either, very skinny build and absolutely no muscle in sight!

While all this sounds funny Richard obviously never had any intentions of coming to work out with me as he wasn't even anywhere near my area! Not really sure if this guy amused me or annoyed me for totally wasting my time. Still, it gave me a laugh and just goes to show people aren't always who or what they claim to be!

27

How much are you going make us this week? …Err, probably nothing!

After several weeks of studying for my personal training certification around the regular jobs I was doing at the time, I had now officially passed the exam, and was now recognized by one of the big name training certification organizations. With certificate in hand I set about finding a gym to work at. With so many gyms around these days, shouldn't be a problem. So I applied at one of the bigger name gyms and was hired immediately. Sadly, it wasn't to be a good experience.

My first taste of being a full time personal trainer in one of the big corporate gyms in the United States lasted all of one day! I was excited to start training people but soon realized their philosophy is more to do with sales than genuinely helping people. Without doubt a case of purely money making and nothing more.

My first red flag concerning this place was during orientation, a two hour briefing about the company, and about personal training that was hosted by the head of human resources, nothing unusual about that of course, but the fact this lady was at least 80lb over weight was kind of shocking to say the least.

She admitted she didn't workout, and proved her ignorance on several occasions by stating facts that clearly were not true about training! It was very obvious everyone in attendance knew she was wrong but no one felt like it was their job to correct her, after all, everyone wants to create a good first impression, and telling the head of human resources that's she's wrong might not go down too well.

Before I could be let loose to train clients they gave me two weeks of training, which was basically nothing more than sales training, after which I felt more equipped to be selling cars or something similar! A little bit of training concerning personal training which was conducted by a kid barely out of school who looked like he'd never even been in a gym before! I was asking him questions that he couldn't possibly answer, his only response being "Let me ask the fitness manager about that question" not too impressed so far you might say.

It was 8.00am Monday morning and I had just signed in for my very first shift after two weeks of extensive training, and within ten minutes a meeting was called in the manager's office-apparently a weekly event-where around twelve trainers were present, in fact I was told by another trainer anyone missing would be subject to disciplinary action, so this must be some serious shit I'm thinking.

The fitness manager, a huge bull of a man clearly on steroids stood clutching his clip board and asked the first trainer how much money he would be making the company this week, the trainer said "Three thousand dollars this week" as he made a note of this the fitness manager replied "Make it four thousand ok" and by the tone of his voice he wasn't asking, rather demanding. After he fired the same question at the first three or four trainers it was very obvious whatever the trainer responded with it wasn't enough. There's a pattern to this bullshit I'm thinking, no matter what I say he`ll demand another thousand dollars on top.

So it`s finally my turn "Nigel, how much are you going to make for the company this week?" My response loud and clear without hesitation was "Err, probably nothing, it`s my first day" everyone in the room burst into hysterical laughter, everyone that is apart from the two managers. The fitness manager frowned saying "See me in my office after please" I already knew this wasn't for me and stood up and said "Forget it, I may as well be a car salesman as be a trainer here" and promptly walked past the two open mouthed astonished managers and straight out the front doors never to return again, and even to this day I absolutely refuse to step foot in this gym. Just the thought of that place leaves a bad taste in my mouth!

Another thing I particularly didn't like was that they encouraged you to interrupt people working out and tell them they are exercising wrong if you see them doing something incorrectly. Sounds fair enough but when the person you tell snaps back saying something like "I've been working out like this for 20 years! Don't tell me I'm training wrong, I know more than you!" It kind of gets old very quickly, and even though my approach was always friendly, it was obvious my interference wasn't welcome at all.

I knew I could make it as a personal trainer on my own without the help of the corporate gyms, and this indeed proved to be the case, sure it's a money making business, what isn't these days? But do they have to make it quite so obvious? I don't think so.

28

Leaving your keys in your pocket can be painful!

Having been working out now for the best part of 30 years I've been fortunate to avoid any serious injuries, especially when you consider I had no idea what I was doing the first few years it's a wonder I didn't cripple myself back then!

So apart from the usual sore muscles and aches and pains, I've escaped any real injuries…Oh, apart from when a little mishap on the leg press resulted in me being unable to walk for 5 weeks! Most injuries usually occur due to lifting too heavy and not performing exercise correctly due to inexperience. But what if you're an experienced personal trainer? Even then freak accidents can happen, read on…Warning, this story isn't for the squeamish!

Its Friday, and it`s leg day. The reason it being leg day is simple it's going to hurt like hell! Plus, it will give me the weekend to recover! After all, how many people do legs on a Monday? Not many as it's not too much fun hobbling around trying to work with legs that won't cooperate. I was expecting some pain afterwards but not quite like the feeling that was coming my way.

After doing various leg exercises such as squats, leg extensions and leg curls it's now time to hit the leg press, my favorite way to finish off the legs is to perform sets of 20 reps starting off with 200lb and ending at 1000lb and coming back down again, 100lb heavier each set till I reach my heaviest set then 100lb lighter till I'm back where I started, get the picture right? I have performed this 'grand finale` hundreds of times without incident. Today however, was going to be different.

For some reason unknown to myself I decided to leave my car keys in my pocket today! Everything was fine until I reach 400lb coming back down- which is only 2 sets away from ending this workout-then disaster strikes! The largest key in my pocket has positioned itself just above my right testicle! And with the help of 400lb behind it the key goes straight into my groin. Now, with my legs being so pumped this doesn't hurt like you'd expect. I kind of figured this isn't a good thing that had just happened, but had no idea the damage that could have just occurred.

At this time I happened to be working a night shift in a local factory, so when I get home I go to bed thinking my sore groin will be ok later when I get up to go to work. When I wake up the pain is incredible! Also very swollen, no work for me tonight. I call in and explain the situation to my supervisor who proceeds to laugh like crazy and asks "Does it hurt?" Maybe its human nature to laugh at other peoples misfortunes when it comes to injury to this delicate area of the body but everyone seems to find this very amusing indeed! I can assure you I didn't find it the least bit funny!

Next morning it's a trip to the Doctor who asks "Does it hurt?" after a quick check down below she sends me on my way to the hospital, and I swear she had something that resembled a smirk on her face! So, now at the hospital my right testicle is doing a very convincing impression of a baseball! That's how big it is now.

A very attractive nurse comes in and puts a rubber glove on and asks "Does it hurt?" while balancing the offending body part carefully in her hand. Then she leaves and is replaced by another pretty nurse who proceeds to do exactly the same thing and of course asks "Does it hurt?" she then says "This is a freak accident" Oh really? No shit! Who would have guessed that! She is replaced by yet another pretty nurse. Now, having your balls held by all these attractive nurses might seem like ecstasy, but considering my delicate injury it's absolute agony!

They take a scan and conclude no serious damage has happened as the key hadn't quite punctured the skin, just very heavy swelling and bruising.

As I'm in no condition to go out at the weekend I call my friend and explain what has happened, he immediately bursts into hysterical laughter and asks "Does it hurt?" Now, I'm not looking for sympathy but a little understanding wouldn't hurt.

For the next few weeks I'm confined to the bed and can only lay on my right side and even the pressure of the bed sheet is excruciating. This is especially hard considering I'm an active person, but now with nowhere to go and nothing to do I'm not a happy camper!

Anyway to cut a long painful story short, I couldn't walk for 5 weeks! After which the swelling finally went down and I returned to work and the gym, but kept a safe distance from the leg press!

Oh, and to answer everyone's question of "Does it hurt?" yes, it fucking hurt like hell!

29

That girl belongs to me…I own her!

Occasionally you meet the strangest, and most unlikely looking couples. People that you can tell just don't belong together at all. I had an email from a couple claiming they want training so we set up a time to come and look around the gym.

When I first met Rita and Bob I immediately thought this was father and daughter as there was obviously a huge age gap. Rita was 33 and Bob was 67 years old. After I gave them the usual guided tour around the gym they agreed they wanted to hire me, actually Bob wasn't interested in training so it was just Rita, I'm thinking he must have just come along for support or perhaps she can't drive, it's possible.

When Rita went to the rest room Bob paid me and he said "This is a lot of money! I expect to see results" I reassured him we would get the results Rita wanted, he said "Good, because this is my girl, I own her!" Now that was a little weird to say the least, I realize this is his daughter but to say he owns her is way over the top. But of course things weren't quite as I thought…

When Rita came for her first session I asked her had her dad brought her to the gym, she laughed and said "Bob is my boyfriend not my dad" she went on to tell me he's way over the top jealous and controlling. I`m thinking probably so considering he already said he owns her! Rita was outstanding during the first session and I couldn't have wished for a better client, one hour after she left I received the following text message that totally shocked me!

"This is Bob, Rita`s boyfriend, how did she do? Just let me know if she gives you any problems, I'll put her straight whatever way it takes, I own this girl and believe me she will do as I say! Or else…"

Or else what? I wouldn't like to think what else. Ok, this is a little worrying to receive this kind of text as it's obvious he has a real hold over Rita, she later tells me he's like her shadow, almost like a stalker! If that's possible to live with someone who stalks you? Guess so, not sure really though, either way it's a strange situation for sure. Anyway I just sent Bob a quick reply telling him how good she did, his reply "Ok, but remember what I said she's mine I own her!" I'm thinking ok Bob, whatever, I get the message!

After a month of very strenuous hard core sessions in which we were making great progress Rita suddenly announced she's taking a month off as she's having a boob job and tummy tuck, all at the expense of Bob no doubt! Kind of disappointing as we were seeing great results. She also tells me he's jealous of her working out with me! Bob obviously is a little insecure to say the least.

After a month I get a text from Rita saying she's almost ready to return to the gym, this is good news I'm thinking as she was one of my best ever clients. Then she tells me there's just one slight problem, she doesn't have any money for training sessions, I tell her I'm sure she could persuade Bob to pay for them like he did before, her reply shocks me! She's just dumped him after he paid for her to have all this surgery! This was her exact reply...

"I dumped that son of a bitch after I had my surgery, couldn't stand him any longer so got what I could out of that old bastard and left him, believe me it's the best thing I've ever done, Bob`s pissed and cleaning his guns so I'm keeping a low profile for a while, I'm staying with friends till this shit blows over"

So I asked her if she feels and looks any better after her surgeries, her reply again is shocking "Well, I was hoping you could check me out and decide if I look any better, I thought we might meet outside the gym if you know what I mean? I think you'll enjoy exploring me, you helped create this new body…I'm all yours!"

Oh, I knew exactly what she meant. Thanks, but no thanks! This girl was obviously nothing more than a gold-digger, I didn't even bother responding especially after she told me Bob was pissed and on the warpath with his collection of guns!

Who in their right mind would get involved in this drama? Not me that's for sure. Sounds like old Bob didn't quite have the control over Rita as he thought he had, what was it he said? "That's girls mine, I own her" whatever Bob, dream on! Thankfully I never did hear from either of them ever again!

30

The client that paid for me to workout!

One thing about being a personal trainer is you have to give the client what they want, even if what they want is a total waste of their money and your time. You know the old saying "The customer is always right" even when they're wrong it seems, which with many of them is pretty often.

A classic example of a client having more money than they know what to do with was Tara who requested the 8pm time slot, as this time was free I gave it her. She claimed she just wanted to tone up and improve her overall fitness. As she claimed she was already in shape I expected a pretty easy training session, I didn't quite expect it to be this easy though.

As we warmed up on the treadmill she asked would it be ok to change the channel on the TV as her favorite program was on. No problem, as there was never anyone else in the gym at this time, I changed it over for her. Whatever it takes to make them feel more comfortable, as it turned out Tara got very comfortable, actually to the point of not doing anything at all!

After 5 minutes I asked her if she was ready to really start the session, her reply amazed me as she said "No I'm fine, you go ahead and workout if you want, I want to watch my program" I wasn't quite sure if she was joking or not to start with, so I just laughed, but she was very serious.

So basically she's paying good money for me to work out while she walks very slowly on the treadmill watching her favorite program on TV, She even used to bring coffee so she could relax and enjoy her show! She would walk very slowly for a few minutes then stop completely to stand on the treadmill and watch her show!

After several weeks her favorite program had come to the end of its current season and so did Tara, she quit, and then returned a few months later for the next season. It was the same thing again, her only interest was in watching TV.

Not that I was complaining, but out of interest I asked her why she couldn't do this at home, she said she didn't have a treadmill at home, I pointed out the fact it would have been way cheaper for her to buy a treadmill than keep paying me full price for nothing. She said "Oh, that's ok, I like working out with you" that made me laugh as she never did a single thing with me. She also said the atmosphere in the gym was more productive than at home! Productive for what? How much motivation does someone need to do absolutely nothing?

Of course she never did get any fitter, and considering she wasn't paying me for that reason it's hardly surprising really! But she did get to watch her favorite TV program and I got paid for doing nothing.

Both client and trainer were quite content with this unusual arrangement. Maybe if you have money to burn it's no big deal, but I'm not so sure too many people would waste their money like this…or maybe they would?

31

Another client that paid for me to workout!

Yet another generous client who paid for my services but never used them like he should have done was a guy named Allan, he came to me wanting to improve his endurance as he was a long distance runner. Allan was very lean and in very good shape. Should be pretty easy I'm thinking, once again, I didn't expect it to be this easy!

The day of the first session arrived, Allan stretched for 5 minutes then asked would it be ok if he went for a short run around the block to get warmed up, I said sure just don't expect me to come too as I'm no runner, just not for me at all, not something that interests me, just not built for it I guess. But, each to his own as they say.

Anyway, so off he went, I'm expecting maybe 10 minutes and he`ll be back but as I can see him out of the gym window running past the first block, he's disappearing way into the distance, I'm thinking just how far is he thinking of going? Obviously his idea of a warm up and mine are a little different. Slight understatement there!

15 minutes passes and no sign of Allan, so I start to work out myself, may as well do something productive while my client is on the run! Then 30 minutes passes and still no sign! Now I'm thinking maybe he's been in an accident or something. Finally after 50 minutes he's back in the gym doing his stretching again, this time to cool down. By this time the full hour is up and he says "great session, I enjoyed that, see you next time" and off he went seemingly very content with what he's just paid good money for. Each to his own, but I certainly

wouldn't pay a trainer that kind of money then go running the streets the full hour! I wouldn't even pay me to do that!

This went on for 2 months, twice a week. This guy would pay me basically to come into the gym to stretch as part of his warm up, then take off running, and return back 50 minutes later to stretch to cool down, and then go home! A little eccentric to say the least.

I just used his hour to workout myself as he obviously didn't need me for anything at all. I didn't even bother to question why he felt the need to pay a trainer to go running by himself. He was happy with this strange arrangement and I certainly didn't mind getting paid for doing nothing.

So, he finally quit after 2 months but I still see him to this day running around the streets, maybe it's time to get him back in the gym for that special stretching again that he used to like to pay me for or maybe he finally figured out he didn't need to pay a trainer to go running by himself!

I miss having a client pay for me to work out while they go running around the streets the full hour! So if you feel like doing this yourself just let me know! I won't object…Honestly!

32

It`s official… I'm the Devil!

Every so often you get a client who really is fun to train even though you know they aren't really taking the training seriously, certainly where diet is concerned, and one that you know probably won't stay too long, but having said all that they still manage to light up the whole gym with their wonderful personality.

One new client who we will call Sheila came to me weighing in at 400lb and naturally wanting to lose weight. Sheila was a perfect example of this type of popular fun client. She claimed she had tried every diet under the sun, but nothing worked! Now if I had a dollar for every time I've heard that from clients I'd probably be well on the way to being a millionaire by now! So from experience I knew she hadn't really put too much effort into all the diets she claimed to have tried.

She really tried her best and worked out as hard as she possibly could, which sadly wasn't too hard, but at least she did try. She spent most of the session screaming and reciting scripture very loudly! Also screaming about the food she could be eating instead of training. She was a very nice and funny lady who soon became great entertainment for everyone who happened to be training at the same time in the gym. The type of person you just couldn't help but like as she generated such a fun atmosphere.

As she worked out at 6am she would still be eating her breakfast in the car as she drove up which suspiciously looked like McDonalds! Not exactly ideal preparation for a training session, her screaming would wake up the gym owner who wasn't an early riser. He came running out panicking thinking the place was on fire or something! She came in with her hair permed and left with it straight as she sweat so much during her sessions.

She would be screaming "Lord, please protect me from this devil I am paying to torture me" and "Lord, what I have I done that was so bad to justify me deserving this evil treatment!" also another favorite of hers was "I could be home eating fried chicken but instead choose to pay this devil to torture me, the Lord works in mysterious ways for sure, Amen" much to the amusement of everyone in the gym.

She paid for 20 sessions and to her credit she did use them all and never missed one single session, not many can say that. but sadly she didn't renew claiming it was costing too much to fix her hair three times a week after each session, so chose to quit at that stage, she also had car trouble so that didn't help matters either.

I heard from Sheila occasionally a few years ago threatening to come back and fight the devil in the gym again….me! But so far she hasn't come back, we shall see, maybe one day. If so, she will be a welcome return.

33

Client needs a reduction in the size of her…What??

Once a client gets used to you and takes you into their confidence you can never be quite sure what they might ask you, or indeed show you as this client did one night.

I had been training Tina for a few years and with great results to show for her years of hard work. She first came to me around 50lb over weight, I got her weight down and looking nicely toned, and she was enjoying her new look, until one day she decided a certain part of her body needed some special attention!

I figured I was being hit on here because her gym attire was getting a little more revealing over the last few weeks, and her personality and actions were starting to get a little flirty too, she seemed to be purposely bending over in front of me every chance she got, which was something she`d never done before. Maybe she was enjoying showing off her new body a little too much now.

Near the end of one session she asked me very shyly if she could ask me a question about training, I thought this was kind of odd really as that's part of my job to answer training questions that a client may want to know about. She said she was very happy with her overall new look apart from one area. This is when I knew she was interested in me and not just showing off her body. Unfortunately for her I didn't feel the same way towards her. However, I wasn't quite prepared for her next move.

As I trained her late at night no one else was in the gym, she suddenly dropped her shorts revealing nothing underneath saying "What exercises can I do to reduce the size of my pussy?" Not sure what shocked me most, the fact she had dropped her shorts in front of me or the ugly part of her body she had revealed! After a quick look I said "I think you better see a surgeon, there's nothing I can do with that sorry" She looked almost offended and quickly pulled back up her shorts. We carried on training for the last ten minutes of the session in silence. She then quickly left without saying anything.

I started getting emails with photos of Tina in sexy underwear, I pretended not to know anything about them and never mentioned them the next time I saw her. So, she stepped up her game plan, the next night I got several emails from Tina with close up photos of her ugly body part!

Ok time to put a stop to this pretty quickly I'm thinking. I responded by telling her could she use a better camera as these photos were pretty bad! That did the trick! She got the message I wasn't interested in her, and never sent me anymore emails containing revealing photos.

Unfortunately she never came back to the gym either, probably too embarrassed or too angry to return, maybe both? I always wondered did she ever get that thing taken care of. Not by me she didn't anyway.

34

The crazy gym dog that put the whole block out!

During this particular week the weather had been very stormy with very strong winds causing quite a bit of damage. During the night the wind had brought down some power lines outside the gym causing a temporary power failure, not such a big deal as it was only 5am and my first client wasn't due until 6am, and with the electric company already working on the issue it should be business as usual, or so I thought.

The electric company had been very busy restoring power lines all throughout the area during the night and were soon busy outside the gym. They said it was only a 5 minute job repairing this problem. The electric worker was trying very carefully to replace some item high up on top of the phone pole by using a 20ft pole with a hook on the end of it.

The guy who owned the gym was outside with his dogs while they went about their early morning business. One of the dogs in particular was very high energy and couldn't stand still for more than a few seconds without getting into something.

All the time the gym owner was talking to the electric worker making it difficult for the guy to concentrate on the task. He said if he made contact with the live wires it would cause more damage than ever, and most likely put the whole block out!

After a few unsuccessful attempts he thought he had got it this time, just as this dog came charging across the parking lot and jumped up pushing the guy over causing the pole to fly out of his hand and hit the live wire! The result of which was an enormous blue flash that ran the entire length of the wire causing a total black out of the whole area!

The gym owner quickly disappeared with the offending dog and drove off in his car and wasn't seen again for quite a few hours. The electric worker was quite shaken but not hurt, but wasn't too happy to say the least as he now knew what should have been a 5 minute job was going to take hours to fix thanks to that crazy dog.

By the time my first client came it was already light outside, we just left the gym door open to let some air in and it was business as usual. It took the electric company the rest of the morning to fix this problem, during which time the gym owner called me leaving a message to call him when they had gone, which I did and like magic he suddenly appeared laughing like crazy about what had happened.

The dog was a constant pain in the ass, as the owner let it roam freely around the gym. Not everyone wants a dog licking them while they're on the ground doing sit-ups, or snarling at everyone that walks through the door, especially when they happen to be new clients, doesn't exactly create a good first impression.

Sadly though, this particular dog was stolen from outside the gym one day the week after this incident and never returned. The only witness who saw this happen from a distance claimed someone took the dog in a truck that looked very similar to a truck used by the electric company, but wasn't positive about this, with no proof nothing could be done.

I wonder if it was the same electric worker guy who got zapped that morning getting revenge by stealing the dog. Probably so!

35

Don't eat fried chicken before kickboxing!

Probably one of the hardest parts of being a personal trainer is the constant battle we have of trying to get clients to avoid eating junk food. We can advise clients on eating correctly, but can't force them to choose their food wisely, so basically, we can only control what happens inside the gym.

Outside the gym is a different matter altogether, the client themselves must show some discipline and self-control with their eating habits, calories in versus calories out, it's that simple, sounds simple enough but certainly not easy, having said that you wouldn't expect someone to eat fried chicken one hour before a kickboxing session! Would you?

Recently my client Jane had been experiencing a lack of energy towards the end of her sessions, as kickboxing is a very demanding workout I suggested she ate something such as oatmeal one hour before she worked out. This is light but also filling and would give her the energy to see this session through till the end. She said it sounded like a good idea and would give it a try.

So, next session Jane comes well prepared confirming she did indeed eat an hour earlier, I asked if she'd had oatmeal as I had suggested, she very quietly whispered "yes" unable to look at me while she said that, so I pretty much knew she wasn't being truthful, the body language gives it away every time you know. If someone can't look you in the eyes, that tells you everything.

Anyway all was well until 20 minutes into the session, when she suddenly turns a very pale color and starts sweating heavily and feeling dizzy, I'm just about to ask if she wants to take a break for a few minutes as she isn't looking too well at all when all of a sudden I hear this almighty retching sound, followed by an ugly sounding large splash! She has just emptied the entire contents of her stomach down the full length of the kicking bag!

By the looks of the chunks that are sliding down the bag I know for sure whatever she ate for breakfast wasn't oatmeal! She confessed that it was actually fried chicken she ate! She didn't have any oatmeal in the house but did have fried chicken so that's what she ate. That says it all really, someone that has fried chicken in the house but not oatmeal isn't really serious about their diet at all.

As her punishment for being so stupid she was made to clean the mess up and wipe down the kicking bag thoroughly, or be fired for lying to her trainer! Luckily she was the last of my kickboxing clients that particular day, so with the windows open overnight the bag was as good as new the following day, well, almost.

The incident was quickly forgotten and Jane remains one of my best clients. She quickly got rid of the fried chicken and equally as fast stocked up on plenty of oatmeal, her energy level was quickly at an all-time high and she continues to go from strength to strength in the gym. I do love a story with a happy ending!

36

The overweight doctor who couldn't follow his own advice!

One of the biggest and most common of problems is getting clients to stay on a healthy diet, after all, why waste money on a trainer if you're going to ruin the whole thing by eating junk food? Doesn't make sense really. A classic example of a client not following a healthy diet happened to be a doctor who specialized in weight loss surgery! Hard to believe, right?

The doctor in question is David, he contacted me claiming he needed to lose a lot of weight. I set up a time for him to come down to the gym to look around and meet me, then decide if he`d like to sign up for some training sessions. At this time of course I had no idea he was a doctor. He tells me this little detail when I meet him, and is concerned his patients won't take him seriously when he's advising them about weight loss. After all, would you take advice from someone who is heavier than yourself concerning weight loss? No, of course you wouldn't. So his fear was well founded.

It was very interesting chatting to him about weight loss, he goes on to tell me that most people who come to him are looking for the easy option rather than actually even trying a healthy diet. He also tells me he only believes in this kind of surgery when all else has failed and it's a matter of life and death to the person concerned. Before he will even agree to consider any weight loss surgery he advises and recommends certain steps to try to avoid this. Listening to him, he clearly understands this whole thing, but can't do it himself it seems. This is without doubt one of the strangest situations I've dealt with so far during my years as a personal trainer.

He believes weight loss surgery isn't the answer for the average person who is looking for a quick fix, simply because he doesn't believe it changes the way people think about food. He says people must train themselves to realize they don't need to be eating all day long. Now that's kind of funny coming from a guy who clearly doesn't follow his own advice! He goes on to admit his weakness is chocolate and will easily consume up to 10 bars a day!

He continues "I really try to make them the understand the importance of diet and exercise, and that they really need to consult with a nutritionist and personal trainer who can both help them without resorting to surgery. I believe as a country the United States is literally eating itself to death with no signs of this ending anytime soon. We must stop people from seeing food as their comfort cushion, like the saying goes eat to live not live to eat, so you see Nigel, I really need to lose the weight to add any credibility to my words" this guy seems to be genuinely nice, so I feel sorry for him and promise to help get the weight off him as by this stage he's already committed to buying 20 sessions to start with.

He says he gives the patient a three month time frame in which to show they are serious about trying to lose weight by recommending a structured diet, sadly he went on to explain only around 30% follow this, he says everyone seems to have some kind of comfort food or drink that they aren't willing to cut out, such as chocolate, fried food, beer and wine etc. he confirms he likes all those comfort foods! This might not be so easy, I know from experience when someone had these kind of addictions it's very difficult to break the habit of a lifetime.

And so it proved to be the case, as David trained with me for a total of 6 months regularly, but with very little weight loss to show for his efforts. It just wasn't meant to be as he couldn't control what he was eating. He claimed he never felt better but eventually he lost interest and gave up altogether.

I hear from him occasionally from time to time threatening to make a comeback, but I highly doubt it will happen. He will just settle for being the overweight doctor who continues to advise people on weight loss that sadly can't follow his own advice.

37

Massage therapist with no happy ending for anyone!

One particular morning I had a call from a lady enquiring about personal training sessions, she asked if I'd be interested in exchanging training sessions for massages. As much as I enjoy a good massage, I turned this offer down as I don't do exchanges. As this is my only job, I would rather just get paid than start exchanging. No sense in cutting your own profits down. She was still interested and thought my prices were reasonable, so we arranged a time for her to start her training.

When I first met Debbie she seemed like any other client who was very eager to improve her fitness level, she claimed she was a massage therapist, but seemed very vague about answering any questions I asked about this profession. At the time I just put it down to her not wanting to talk about her job too much. I mean, not everyone wants to talk about their job in their spare time away from it, nice to have a break occasionally and forget about work so I didn't really think any more about it.

Anyway, everything was going fine after about 2 months of regular training in which time Debbie had made great progress, and really was proving to be one of my best clients. She could do it all, from weights and kickboxing to self-defense. Nothing seemed to phase this girl. She was good fun too, always dancing around between the rounds when we kick boxed. Not sure if this was her way of showing me she didn't need to take advantage of the break or maybe she was practicing some other mysterious moves associated with her profession.

Things all changed the day she turned up very drunk one morning! Considering she worked out at 9am I thought it very strange that she should be so drunk so early, must be a story behind this I thought, and there certainly was....

After being so reluctant to talk about her job she suddenly went into great graphic detail about her mysterious profession. Turns out she wasn't a massage therapist at all... but a hooker! She had been hard at work all night and decided to celebrate before her training session! She spent the entire hour telling me in great detail about her busy nights work, including her specialty of taking two men at once! And her 'happy endings' massages!

After an hour of graphic detail, she claimed she wasn't feeling too good and would reschedule her training session later in the week. She made a call for a friend to pick her up and staggered out of the gym, I had a feeling that was going to be the last time I would see Debbie at the gym, and sadly that proved to be the case.

I can only imagine how embarrassed she must have been when she realized just exactly what she had told me in her drunken state! She never responded to my emails or calls, so all in all not such a happy ending...I lost a good client!

About a year later I did bump into Debbie in a local gas station, I was just leaving as she was walking in, she put her head down and pretended not to notice me. Oh well, still embarrassed I guess. I didn't bother to ask if she wanted to come back training again.

38

The dangerous new client!

One of the best ways of attracting new clients is through training one of their friends who then recommends your services, that way they already have confidence in your ability and know you can do the job as they've already seen the results, so you can't beat a word of mouth referral, here is an example of this, and a very unusual occurrence along with it.

One of my regular clients told me he knew a young lady who he worked with that was interested in starting training with me, she was impressed by the changes she had seen in him over the months. So after a few emails we worked out a time that would suit her and we set up her first session.

My client called me laughing, and warning me this girl had an interesting experience a couple of days before her first session, but was a very shy girl and wouldn't tell me as it was very personal. Well, I thought if it was so personal I don't need to know anyway! I really don't need to know everything my clients are doing away from the gym.

After greeting my new client Sarah, a very fit looking 28 year old Mexican lay, we started warming up on the treadmill for a few minutes. She seemed to be very shy and nervous, just like my client had told me she was. With this being early on a Monday morning I happened to ask her how was her weekend. I thought this would be a good way of getting her to open up and feel more comfortable, I wasn't quite prepared for her response!

With a very mischievous grin on her face, my new client took great delight in telling me how she broke her boyfriend's dick at the weekend! Then went into great detail about how he was taking her from behind when she suddenly thrust backwards with great force and that's when the damage was done! So much for her being shy I thought.

She went on to tell me how the poor man spent most of the weekend in the emergency room resulting in a very delicate operation in a very delicate area. She then went on to say she had dumped him, adding "What use is a man with a broken dick to a girl? None at all!" I didn't respond.

I've heard about this rare and freak accident happening before, I think I saw a documentary on TV about it, but it was shocking to hear from a new client on her very first session! All within the first 10 minutes of meeting her! I guess that's why it's called personal training! Very personal indeed!

Next day I trained my client who had originally told me about her, I reminded him that it was he who had told me how shy this girl was. He burst out laughing saying "She's crazy, so how long did it take her to tell you the story?" I told him she had told me within the first 10 minutes of meeting her, he said "Oh yes, that sounds just like my little sister, like the little whore that she is!"

39

The dog that made my client lose her hair!

Walking on the treadmill can be pretty boring but can also be a good source of entertainment people watching, you get to see things otherwise you might miss, especially when the treadmills are next to the wall, and facing the entire gym.

One particular morning I was walking on the treadmill waiting for my next client to arrive when I noticed a little dog scooting across the gym floor on its butt leaving a trail of shit behind it! The dog belonged to another trainer's client, not mine. It looked kind of funny at first, but when I noticed it had crapped on the gym floor that wasn't so amusing.

The mess was quickly cleaned up by the dog's owner, I'm sure she thought no one had noticed but I had a perfect view of the whole incident. I pretended to be texting on my phone as she looked very embarrassed. She cleaned it up so I thought that's fair enough, no need to say anything.

My client came soon after and I quickly forgot about what I had just witnessed, the offending dog's owner left the gym soon after the incident, along with the guilty dog of course. Anyway, the next day all these little worm like things were wriggling around the gym floor where the dog had been, I noticed each day they seemed to be getting more and more of them, and not content with staying in this particular area they were now taking over the whole gym floor! It may have been a coincidence, but the owner of the gym had just recently had a new carpet fitted and figured that's where they had come from, I wasn't so sure about that though.

One week later my client Mary, a big black lady with a afro hairstyle was finishing her workout with a few minutes of sit-ups on the ground, when I noticed these little worms wriggling their way over to her, several managed to creep into her hair! I was too shocked and horrified to say anything to her as I stared in disbelief at what I was seeing!

Mary was working out of town the following week, so it was two weeks later that I saw her next, when she walked into the gym she looked very different and very embarrassed, actually wearing a baseball cap, at first I thought she must have got a different hairstyle, in a way she had but it wasn't through choice, I was trying my best not to stare at her new look too much, but something wasn't quite right about her appearance.

When she removed her cap it looked like someone had totally chopped off most of her hair! She went on to explain that the day after our last training session, her head began to severely itch resulting in large clumps of her hair falling out, to the extent that she was now half bald! By coincidence she had started using a new shampoo around the time of the incident with the dog and put it down to a severe reaction to this new shampoo.

Severe reaction indeed! Most likely from the dog shit & worms, and not from the new shampoo!

40

The client who wanted to be taller!

You never really know what to expect when you meet a client for the first time, sometimes it's good, sometimes bad, and then again sometimes it's just plain weird! This clients request was about as weird as they come.

On this particular day I was meeting with a potential new client, not an actual training session, but rather just to show him around the gym and discuss what his fitness goals might be, and basically let him decide if he wanted to hire me as his trainer. After all, there's so many trainers out there these days you may as well pick one you feel comfortable with, that's why I give them the chance to check it all out first.

Ray was a very short stocky guy standing 5 feet tall and weighing in at 250lb which didn't exactly give him a very balanced look at all. Ray claimed his biggest problem was his lack of motivation to work out by himself and of course his diet, he knew what he should and shouldn't be eating but found it very difficult to stick to a diet, sounds familiar I'm thinking. If I had a dollar for every time I have heard this all too familiar story I would be a very rich man indeed.

He seemed to be quite knowledgeable about the training and diet, so I thought I could probably really help him as he was very enthusiastic about getting some help. If a client comes with the right attitude and is willing to listen then it makes results so much easier to achieve.

So, after talking in depth about my training program he figured I would be a good trainer for him. Great! I got a new client, at the end of our meeting I asked Ray what he would most like to achieve from working out with me, I was expecting to hear the usual request of dropping a few pounds and tone up etc. To my amazement though, Ray said "I would really like to be 6 inches taller, what can we do about that?" Err, let's see now, how about nothing I'm thinking!

Strange thing was he wasn't even joking! "How the hell am I supposed to make you taller?" I asked him. No response was his reply, so I suggested he start wearing bigger boots! I was joking of course, but he seemed to take this seriously adding if he was a woman high heels would work great, and maybe he should consider becoming a cross-dresser! As he said that I'm looking at him hoping to see or hear some sign of that being a joke, but there wasn't any, he was serious.

I was more shocked when he got out his check book, and that he actually decided to still want to hire me or any trainer! He paid for twenty sessions but never did start training with me. Money for nothing! Oh well, no complaints from me. I have no idea whatever happened to this guy. Maybe he had a reality check and realized just how crazy his request was.

I swear some people think hiring a trainer is like hiring a magician! We just wave this magic wand and they get anything they want, but when their request is as crazy as this one not even a magician can help, let alone a personal trainer.

41

The naughty night nurse!

Many people come to the gym straight from work, so it's quite a common sight to see clients carrying a sports bag or some other type of bag with a change of clothes inside, or something else altogether inside. Something that might have been forgotten about was still inside that bag, and should probably be at home safe and sound, and unseen by gym members or anyone else for that matter.

Karen was a very attractive young nurse and came to work out at 7am straight from her night shift at the local hospital. She had been coming training regularly for 3 months without fail, and although she was naturally very flirty, it was all good natured without incident until this particular morning. That was about to change big time!

The gym was steadily filling up as around 5 or 6 trainers had clients at this time. As usual Karen came walking into the gym with a change of clothes in a bag, this time though the bag slipped out of her grip as she caught it on the edge of the leg press machine, the bag was already open resulting in a very large black object falling out of her bag and rolling across the gym floor, none other than the biggest vibrator you could ever imagine!

This thing was enormous! With it being perfectly round it rolled half way across the gym floor and came to rest right in front of the row of treadmills, as this spectacle was seen by around 20 people there was no trying to hide the fact what it was and who it belonged to. No one was watching the TV any longer as a much more interesting and entertaining situation was developing right in front of them!

I couldn't help but look at the expressions on people faces. The younger people in the gym were laughing, the middle-aged people were trying not to laugh, while the elder ones were in total shock! I heard one elderly lady mutter to her workout partner "What on earth does she do with one that size?" her friends response "I can't imagine, but it makes my eyes water just thinking about it!" I was laughing to myself at this stage.

But Instead of being embarrassed, with all eyes watching her every move Karen calmly walked over to where this thing had rolled over to, picked it up and gave it a good shake in front of all the disbelieving eyes and said "Come back here you!

This is my good friend Fred, I`d better go and wash him now as I'll need him later" which she did, then calmly came back without a care in the world and casually walked over to her gym bag drying Fred off with a towel saying "That's better, you're all nice and clean again, now you stay where you belong you hear me!" it sounded like she was talking to a dog or something!

She said to me "That was funny wasn't it" what was even funnier was the reaction to this classic moment by other people in the gym, shock and horror mostly! We carried on with the training session like nothing had happened and the incident was never mentioned ever again, although I must admit every time I saw her afterwards that incident never failed to pop into my mind.

It was definitely one of the funniest incidents ever in the gym, and she was definitely the naughty night nurse that morning! And I suspect most mornings and nights too judging by what fell out of her bag!

42

The 20 minute client!

Quite often you come across the type of client who has more money than sense, who sees having a personal trainer as nothing more than a status thing. Perhaps it's a sign amongst the wealthy that they have money to be able to tell their friends that they can afford a trainer. After all, this isn't a cheap service by any means.

Maybe they think it impresses people to bring it up in a conversation "My trainer said this, my trainer said that" which is fine, but when they put no effort in and don't look any different after several months of training it's not a very good advert for your business when they're telling everyone who their trainer is. What trainer in their right mind would want their name associated with someone who isn't getting results? Especially when the client is the one to blame for lack of results, by not putting effort in, or not eating correctly. It does happen... Quite often!

So when they're out and about socializing with their friends, and happily telling everyone who has trained them, their friend's first reaction will probably be something like "Well, he can't be a very good trainer as you still look the same!" Or "What a waste of money! You need a refund!"

So as you can clearly see, that can be a big problem. After all, each client is a walking representative of your training skills, so it pays to have them looking their best as of course it can lead to more business, easier said than done with some though, as it requires them to do their part too.

Dianne was such a client, very nice lady who obviously had money and wasn't too concerned about wasting it. She first came to me with an all too familiar request, that of wanting to lose quite a few pounds. She was in pretty good shape, especially considering the fact she was 60 years old.

So we arranged her first session, it was very apparent when she showed up that she wasn't really into it. For her it was more of a social thing, just having somewhere to hang out for an hour. Each session would end exactly the same way with her constantly looking at the clock, no matter what we were doing, each session would end after only 20 minutes!

With no cool down or anything, she would say "OK, I'm done, great session, thank you, see you next time" and walk out of the gym, this went on for around a year before she must have finally got so bored with it she quit, or maybe she found something else more interesting to occupy her time with.

Easy money for a me of course, as she's still paying for the full hour, but with her choosing only to complete 20 minutes of every session I never had a chance to improve her fitness. Just a case of take the money and don't worry about it, she obviously wasn't so why should I?

She never did come back, although she actually referred several people to me saying I was a great trainer, that's very nice of her to say, but I don't think she could ever honestly say she found that out. Kind of hard when the session lasts only 20 minutes!

43

One rep too many, not a good idea!

One of the most common questions as a personal trainer I get asked is which is better, free weights or machines? Depending on what you're wanting to achieve both have their advantages. All gyms nowadays have both to choose from, and especially very high-tech machines that seem to cover anything you could think of doing in a gym. But what about in the early 80`s when you didn't have the luxury of such things? Homemade equipment, that's what!

One of the first gyms I worked out at was basically an old garage converted into a very rough looking gym, complete with homemade weights! One example would be the Lat-pulldown machine which was nothing more than a bamboo pole for a bar and a steel bucket full of bricks! Not easy to control a swinging bucket, but you know what? It worked! Years later when I worked out in a modern hi-tech gym I was always amazed at how much weight I could handle on this particular exercise, I'm pretty sure all those years controlling the swinging bucket had something to do with it.

Anyway, with this place being an old garage there was no reception or anything else really, just a room full of weights and homemade equipment. Every member had their own key and would let themselves in whenever they wanted to work out. With this garage being in an industrial estate there were no local residents within ear shot to complain about people screaming and shouting and throwing weights around at all hours of the day or night.

At the time I was working a night shift at a local factory so a few work colleagues and myself would go straight to the gym at 6am most mornings. Very rarely was anyone in there working out at that time, but one particular day we unlocked the gym to find someone already in there in a very uncomfortable situation to say the least!

The first thing we see is a guy on the bench press with the bar stuck over his throat! He`s laid there not moving at all with his face bright purple! My friend immediately said "Shit! He`s dead, let's go!" before I could respond a muffled and very distraught voice screamed "Come back! Don't leave me you bastards! Help! Please help me!"

Realizing this guy is still very much alive, we rushed over to the bench and pulled the 200lb bar off the guy's throat and placed it back on the stand, and as we did so, the guy rolled off the bench onto the floor coughing and choking, and thrashing about like a fish out of water!

After a few minutes he had recovered and composed himself enough to explain what had happened, after first thanking us. Apparently it was chest day, and he had been having a great session until he got a little too ambitious, and decided to do one extra set with this 200lb bar when disaster struck! Although it was a weight he could handle easily enough he pushed himself a little too far, resulting in his arms totally giving out, and with no one spotting him, or indeed no one else in the gym he was stuck there with the bar across his throat praying for someone to rescue him.

I'm not saying we saved this guy's life, but certainly saved him from possible injury as no one else came to work out that morning while we were in there. We carried on using this gym at the same early time another 6 months before finding another gym, we never did see that guy ever again.

This story carries a very serious warning, if you're training by yourself with free weights be very careful with exercises such as the bench press, if your arms suddenly give out like this guy, you could find yourself in the same situation. A very dangerous situation indeed.

44

The happy, singing religious family!

One particular night when the phone rang, I could never have imagined what I would hear upon answering it! It was a woman singing some song, not quite sure what the song was, or indeed who the woman was either, as she never said anything at all, only sang! But it sounded interesting enough to hold my attention, so I carried on listening.

Whatever the song was she sang the whole thing, at least 3 minutes of it! When she finished there was a sudden round of applause and cheering in the background, she then sked "What did you think to that?" I said "It was very impressive, but I think you have the wrong number sorry" her response surprised me "Oh no, I have the right number Nigel, and I want you train my whole family"

After finally introducing herself, and various family members, she went on to explain that a total of 8 people wanted training, and could I split them up into maybe 2-3 groups, money wasn't an issue so however I could do it they were in! The bottom line was that they wanted training, and I was the trainer they wanted to train them. We arranged a time for her to come and check the place out, and she said "We won't be boring, I can promise you that!" something told me I think she's right about that.

To start with, all 8 came to look around the gym together. It was quite an entrance into the gym as all of them walked in singing, with the lady who had been singing down the phone on lead vocals, who was in top form, and singing very loudly! Funny thing was the singing went on for ten minutes before anyone even said anything! It was different for sure, but great entertainment.

After the song had finished they all introduced themselves one by one, the father was the one paying for all this, and being a retired bank manager said it wouldn't be a problem, and to emphasize this he already had his check book in one hand and a pen in the other! So after briefly showing them around the gym they quickly decided who wanted to workout with who, and arranged themselves into two groups of four. They seemed happy with this arrangement and as they left the gym they burst out into another song!

My schedule at this particular time was pretty busy, so the only way I could accommodate this whole family was to train the two groups back to back, I had a block of two hours free in the evening, so as one group finished the other group started.

As soon as all 8 saw each other they'd greet one another like old friends reuniting after years apart, and chat enthusiastically about their day, and then instantly burst into song. After the greetings and singing was over, there wasn't too much of the training session left!

This family were all great fun, but all so hyper it was impossible to train them productively. They quit coming after 3 months claiming they couldn't afford it any longer. Sadly, the only thing that improved was their singing!

45

I want to lose 50lb without sweating or breaking a nail!

As a personal trainer you get to meet so many people with such unrealistic expectations regarding what they're wanting to achieve from their training sessions. Even more unrealistic of course when they aren't prepared to do their part. This isn't a magician you're paying! I can't wave a magic wand and you suddenly lose weight! Doesn't work that way unfortunately. You must do your part. Firstly, by showing up regularly and working out hard, I can only show you, but I can't do it for you. Secondly, you must eat correctly, I can only advise you, but I can't force you to make the right choices when it comes to your eating habits.

One of the best examples of this issue was when Sandy showed up. She had emailed me a few days before we set up the first session, she worked as a beautician and really looked the part, very pretty lady indeed. She claimed she needed to lose 50lb, I would say possibly 20lb at most really.

I noticed she was dressed like a model with no other clothes with her, so asked her had she just finished work, her response shocked me when she told me no, she`d actually took the day off today so she would be rested and prepared for our first session!

On one hand she sounds like she's taking this seriously by taking the day off in preparation for her first session, but on the other hand she then shows up for a training session looking like a model about to do a fashion shoot or something! Something just doesn't add up here at all.

When I asked her in detail exactly what she wanted to achieve Sandy said she really wanted to lose 50lb, then shocked me by saying "I don't want to sweat and mess my hair up, or break my nails" as if to emphasize this she waved her immaculately manicured nails in front of me! Ok, so this is going to be a problem, how do you lose 50lb without sweating? Surgery is perhaps her best option!

As she'd already wrote a check out for 20 sessions I wasn't about to tell her that though, after all, business is business, whether they take it seriously or not I still have a living to make here.

I knew instantly this wasn't going to work when she told me the only shoes she had were the high heels she was wearing! She chose the bare foot option, this negative feeling I had was confirmed after a 5 minute warm up on the treadmill, at low speed I might add that probably wasn't even worthy of the title warm up! Sandy was fanning herself every few seconds saying "I had no idea it was going to be this hard, I'm tired out already" I'm stood there thinking you've got to be kidding me, this is only a warm up for God's sake!

To my disappointment, Sandy chose to attend every training session dressed the same way! Nice on the eyes as she was, there's no way I can train someone effectively who comes dressed in this manner, and every time she felt one drop of sweat forming on her brow she would immediately stop exercising and wipe herself down!

She never allowed herself to be trained properly, and never gave herself a chance at losing weight, after a few sessions she emailed me thanking me for trying to help her but exercising just wasn't her thing, and she guessed she was just destined to be overweight. With that attitude, I guess she was right!

At least she did achieve 2 out of the 3 requests she told me about on that first session, she didn't sweat, and didn't break a finger nail! As for losing 50lb... Forget it!

46

One legged man's ridiculous request!

Every so often you receive really crazy emails from potential clients who prove they have no idea what they're talking about by the crap they're asking you! But also occasionally, you get a strange request that you're sure is fake, but then after thinking more about it you're not quite sure whether it's genuine or not.

One such request was allegedly from a guy claiming to have one leg who was in serious training for the world hop-scotch contest! This is the exact email that I received…

"Hi, my name is Brian, and I'm a former hop-scotch world champion, I desperately need your help to regain my title back. Slight problem though, I only have one leg now after a car accident, what exercise can I do now to help me improve in this event? Looking forward to hearing back from you, and hopefully you can get me back where I need to be again, thanks so much"

At first I immediately dismissed this email as a joke and simply deleted it. One night after getting home late from the gym I was sat relaxing just browsing through my emails when I noticed another email from the same guy requesting the same thing as before. This time he had a link to a site that told his story. Ok, now I'm intrigued, I had to read this.

After reading this article there's no doubt it, this was a real person who actually made a living making prosthetic limbs! Whether or not it's the same person who sent the email is a different thing altogether. At this stage I'm still thinking this is most likely a practical joke, possibly from another trainer.

Out of curiosity I went along with it, as the email address matched the one in the link to his website I replied asking when he'd like to come to the gym to start training in order to get his world hop-scotch title back.

To my amazement he responded and actually came to the gym, and everything about him and his story was genuine! You would never believe this guy had only one leg, he was more mobile and willing to try almost anything than most clients with two legs! He worked out really hard, and on leg night he actually switched legs to a newer more athletic leg he'd been working on!

I told him that I'd never heard of a world champion hop-scotch contest, he claimed it was a very low key event, like something that would be in an alternative Olympics. I'd never heard of that either, but he did bring me his medal and trophy in to show off. Not really sure if this was a genuine contest or something he had made up, but as this guy seemed very genuine, and was also very pleasant I gave him the benefit of the doubt.

He trained with me for 6 months right up until he flew out to Japan to compete in his competition (or so he claimed) unfortunately I never heard from him ever again so have no idea how he went on in trying to regain his title, maybe it didn't go down too well, who knows? But this remains one of the strangest requests I ever received.

47

Winston the dog needs to lose some `puppy` fat!

Another very strange request, actually possibly the strangest of them all was when a lady called me asking can you train 2 together, I said yes, and I do regularly so it wouldn't be a problem at all. What she didn't tell me was that the other person was actually a dog! She said "I'll see if Winston can make it, he's not been feeling too good lately, but he needs to lose some puppy fat" so we arranged the first session.

When Katie first walked into the gym, I was expecting to see a husband or son, not a dog! With her saying he needs to lose some puppy fat I figured it would most likely be a young kid. She proudly said "Meet Winston" Winston was a bulldog! "He needs to lose a few pounds, like me" well she was right on both counts! But what exactly am I supposed to do for an overweight bulldog? I'm a personal trainer, not a vet!

My brain was on overdrive thinking about this, and I quickly came up with a solution. As this was 9pm and no one else was in the gym I had an idea, we tied Winston to a treadmill, and at very low speed started it up for 30 minutes. Winston took to it immediately and began his exercise program! He would walk for 30 minutes then crash out on the gym floor for 30 minutes and snore like crazy!

The whole session was based around Winston! Katie would spend the first 30 minutes talking about anything, like the main talking point on the news that particular day, or the weather, anything to avoid training. Basically she was nuts! Very nice lady, but totally nuts! It was very obvious listening to the way she talked about Winston, that she considered him human and not a dog! I understand many people consider their dogs as being real family members (which they are) but surely this is taking it a little too far?

Then she would take over the treadmill after Winston had got his 30 minutes in, and walk even slower than Winston had, and keep talking about nothing the whole time! Strange for sure, but she was paying the same rate as two people would pay so it was very easy money for me! As I'd been in the gym most of the day it was nice to finish off the day with an easy session, and it didn't come much easier than training Winston (and Katie).

They came together for 3 months in which time Winston got in pretty good shape, and actually worked out harder than Katie did! He lost 10 pounds and became quite muscular looking once he shed some `puppy` fat, while she lost nothing at all, but was very happy with Winston`s results! They quit coming soon after, as she claimed he had reached his goal!

She did contact me the week after to ask if I could train her friend's dog, a 120lb Rottweiler! Apparently the dog had anger issues and they thought some exercise might help. I politely declined taking on that new client! Never heard from her again so hopefully Winston kept the weight off and stayed in good shape, as for her... well, hopefully she's doing ok too!

48

The young kid who ruined every session!

For me personally, one of the most annoying and irritating situations about personal training is when clients choose to bring their young kids with them during their training sessions. Many claim they can't afford to hire a babysitter and pay for personal training sessions which is understandable, so bring the kids along with them.

Now occasionally you get lucky and the kids will sit still and read a book or watch TV, but with most young kids having very short attention spans, on most occasions they see the gym as a giant playground which leads to chaos as they're constantly running around distracting and disrupting everyone's attention, trashing the gym, and not to mention the safety aspect of running wild like this.

Now the really annoying situation is when the parent of the kids are totally oblivious to their kid's antics! Or chooses not to notice, many have the attitude that it's an hour that they've paid for, and an hour where someone else gets to deal with their kids, while they get a break and workout, namely me the trainer!

One particular couple always brought their young kid with them, he was around 6 years old and a total brat! No other word for it! On the way over to the gym they'd let him drink soda, so by the time the training session started, the sugar had kicked in and the kid was as high as a kite!

I used to dread this session because I knew the kid would be so hyper that he wouldn't allow his parents to workout properly, with him always demanding to be the center of attention they never got anything from the workouts at all. The wife was serious about wanting to get in shape, but the husband wasn't and was quite happy to use the kid's behavior as an excuse not to do anything. The frustration on his wife's face was obvious.

They trained with me over a year with no results, and I'm really surprised they chose to stay that long, but when the husband started complaining about not getting results it`s time for a reality check here!

I very politely pointed out that the young kid is too demanding of their time during the training session, and they're constantly stopping the exercises to pamper his every needs! Basically the young kid won't allow them to work out, and on the rare occasion they actually told him `no` he would throw a temper tantrum until he got his way. It was a disaster! So having said all that, why would they seriously expect to get results?

They were really nice people and agreed with what I said, the husband wasn't really into the training anyway so agreed to stay home with the kid, leaving his wife free to work out without any distractions as before.

She trained with me a further 6 months with great results, sadly, that came to an end when her husband took a different job with hours that didn't give him the time to look after the kid as before, so basically the choice was bring the kid along again, or quit coming altogether. She quit!

49

The silent, uninterested and unmotivated kid!

Quite often you have to deal with people who simply don't want to be there in the gym working out, so why pay for something that you don't want to do, or get any enjoyment from? That would seem a pretty straight forward question you'd think… right? But not so simple when it's a parent paying for their kid who has no desire to workout.

I have faced this frustrating situation on more than one occasion, but the worst case so far I encountered would be this one…

Jimmy senior and Jimmy junior came to see me one day in the gym after we exchanged several emails, immediately you could tell it was a case of the parent wanting it more than the kid himself. Jimmy senior said money wasn't an issue as he believed the money spent now would save on medical bills in later life for Jimmy junior, very sensible thinking, and also very true.

After meeting them I could understand the parents concern as the kid was already a good 50lb over weight, and at only 16 years of age I knew it wouldn't be easy. After all, time in the gym was time he couldn't spend playing his precious video games! The curse of modern day technology, and sadly a very common problem amongst the younger generation these days.

Every session, either the parents or elder sister would bring Jimmy junior to the gym and pick him up an hour later, which was great as there's nothing worse than having an over eager parent watching the kids every move during the training session.

As soon as he walked through the doors he would drape a towel over his head, much the same as a boxer might do after taking a beating in the ring and not wanting anyone to see the damage to his face. This situation of course was very different, here we have a kid with no confidence and basically not even wanting to be there in the first place!

He very rarely spoke, and when he did it was all about video games! Something I have no interest in at all, so it was a very quiet session. I tried my best to reach out to the kid and help him, but it was impossible as it was obvious by him hanging the towel over his head the way he did that he was hiding behind a shield and basically saying I don't want anything to do with you or your training.

Surprisingly enough though, we did go through a very productive patch during the year he trained with me and lost around 20lb, mainly because his parents were strictly monitoring his diet. It was working though.

Sadly, then comes the major turning point that was to be the downfall to his training, the kid turned 18 and passed his driving test, and as he was a `Straight A` student, his parents kept their promise of buying him a car. That's great, except one little thing, now Jimmy junior was mobile and free to eat all the crappy junk food he could ever want, and of course, that's exactly what he did!

As his already fading interest in the gym finally faded altogether, his weight ballooned alarmingly! He was now heavier than when we first started. With his own wheels, and being 18 he was now free to make his own decisions, which sadly didn't include coming to the gym anymore.

His dad sent me a really nice email saying how much he appreciated my help, but now he realized it was down to the kid himself, we all tried to lay a good foundation down but it just simply wasn't enough. A classic case that once again proves you can't make someone do something they don't want to do, even when it's for their own good.

50

A client's wife, and ex-wife fighting in the gym!

People have many different reasons for wanting to get in shape, usually to look and feel better, or perhaps there's a special occasion or event that's coming up such as a wedding or vacation that they need to look their best for. All understandable, and all good reasons to get in shape.

But when one lady wanted to learn self-defense to beat up her ex-husbands new wife, and his new wife wanted to learn self-defense to beat up his ex-wife, well, that was a new one for me. Slight problem was they all trained with me! I figured they'd probably sort this out sooner or later, but I didn't think it would happen in the gym!

Apparently the new wife and ex-wife had known one another years, and there'd always been bad blood between them. The husband in question told me all 3 of them attended the same school and that this was an ongoing feud between the two ladies. So basically, they'd never liked one another before, but when this guy married both of them and dropped one for the other, the bad feeling became pure hatred. Both were Mexican ladies with fierce tempers!

For 3 months I trained all 3 separately, and did a good job of scheduling them all far away from each other's training times as possible. It was interesting watching both the ladies attack the punching bags, which interestingly enough, both named the bags after the other lady! This added an extra spark to the workouts for sure. I reminded them self-defense is about defending yourself, not attacking someone. They both had the same response… They'd let the other throw the first punch then beat the crap out of them, all in self-defense of course, interesting definition of self-defense you might say.

The guy would jokingly ask me who I thought would win in a fight between the two of them, I said it would be hard to separate them as they're both very evenly matched. This was always the main talking point when he came to the gym, and he would build it up like they do with an upcoming big boxing match. All seemed like harmless fun, but I don't think he ever seriously thought it would happen, I know I certainly didn't.

But on one particular night, it did happen… The present wife must have been driving past and noticed the ex-wife's car in the parking lot, and as it was almost 10pm she knew no one else would be around at that time. She came running in, and it was on! Both ladies ripped into one another immediately like wild animals! The language was nasty, and the fighting pretty violent.

As I'm thinking of the best way to intervene before one of them gets killed, the guy who was married to both of them came running in, he figured what his wife's plan was that night and followed her, one of the best decisions he ever made, as now he gets the job of separating these two crazy women and not me!

To my amazement, as he jumped in to break the fight up, both ladies turned on him and absolutely kicked the living shit out of him! He was knocked down and both were on top of him punching and kicking him senseless! I shouted at them to get out of here or I'm calling the cops, and to prove I was serious I had already punched in 911, and held up my phone for them to see with my finger over the call button threatening to make that call.

His wife ripped off her wedding ring and threw it at him saying something quite nasty in Spanish, well, I can't speak Spanish but I figured it wasn't anything nice anyway! As she walked by she gave him one last kick, followed by the ex-wife who spat on him, and also kicked him as she walked past and both walked out of the gym together like the best of friends, leaving him groaning on the floor!

He slowly got up looking very shaken by the sudden attack, mumbling something about he was expecting that and hobbled out of the gym and that was the last I saw of him or his ex-women! No idea what happened to any of them after the big fight.

So, in conclusion to this drama, to answer the guys long running question as to who would win I have no idea, but I seemed to be the real loser as I had instantly lost 3 regular clients, but after what I'd just witnessed that might not be such a bad thing! A little too much drama you might say.

51

The timid client who was scared of her own shadow!

As a personal trainer you can guarantee you will meet and train every kind of personality that exists! Sadly, not all are good of course. One of the most boring and awkward clients came to me wanting to get in shape, and learn kickboxing.

Slight problem though, she was so unenthusiastic about training and never got out of first gear during the training sessions. Even the way she spoke would make you want to fall asleep listening to her one tone boring voice. In fact, everything about this girl was just plain boring!

Linda came to look around the gym, and after a few nervous moments decided she would give it a go. I say nervous moments simply because this gym being an old building, and the fact it was 9pm there were usually one or two creaks to be heard occasionally, not a big deal really and nothing you wouldn't hear in your own home late at night. But for Linda it was very unsettling. I figured this could be interesting as she wanted to work out at the very same time.

She worked out with very little effort, and could never truly relax enough to settle down. Every little noise would lead to her asking "What was that?" and all the time she was looking around like she was expecting to be attacked at any moment!

Linda was a strange one to be honest, she had one tone to her voice which was very slow and very uninteresting no matter what she talked about, which was usually very little! And her actions in the gym were equally as slow and without much effort. Both those things combined lead to a very unproductive and very boring hour.

I was quite relieved when we came to the end of our 20 sessions, as I had a feeling she wouldn't be renewing, that tells you how bad it was for me, the fact I was willing to lose money here! I just couldn't take her any longer.

This was a particular difficult session to get through, and with it being 9pm and having been in the gym all day long it was simply too much to deal with. So just to help matters on the last session I told her I had heard from some new local client that this gym was the scene of a brutal murder hundreds of years ago, and apparently was haunted by a less than friendly ghost, so that could explain the strange noises. I told her all this while pretending to look around nervously as she always did every session expecting to hear more noises. I thought I'd exaggerate it a little for effect!

Well, that did the trick nicely as Linda totally freaked out and couldn't wait to get out of the gym, that's the fastest I'd ever see her move! She left telling me she was busy for the next few weeks but would be in touch soon after to start up again, which of course she never did. Oh well, you win some, and like this story you lose some… Thank God!

52

The couple who loved my training so much they quit!

One thing about this job that never ceases to amaze me is how hard it seems for many clients to tell me they don't want to renew, whether it be for financial or other reasons. Obviously this is a business so as a trainer you want to keep clients as long as possible, but you also have to be realistic enough to understand most people simply don't have the money to keep paying for this service forever.

With the modern age of technology allowing people to text their excuses rather than tell you the truth face to face, It might take you a while, but once you are familiar with the signs it's very easy to know when someone has no intentions of coming back, simply by the way they elaborate with one excuse after another. Just tell the truth, it's really not that hard, and certainly easier than constantly making excuses that get more ridiculous each time.

A classic example of this problem was when I started training a couple, they worked out hard and got great results and claimed they loved my training style so much they realized they now couldn't live without it, it was part of their lives now they said, it's like a drug that we crave they said, we feel so much better because of you they said. Nice words but they soon proved to be just words and nothing more as we approached the end of the package they had paid for.

During their last session I`m expecting a nice check at the end of the hour, but instead they tell me "Did we mention, we`re out of town the next two weeks? But we`ll renew when we return" the way they said it told me that wasn't true, having heard this so many times before I just wished them well and to contact me when they're ready for training again. I had already written them off to be honest.

Of course they never did contact me again, so I thought I'd call their bluff by contacting them after the two weeks were up telling them I was ready to resume our sessions as soon as they were, it was one excuse after another, it was going to be another week, then another and so on. I continued to call their bluff by contacting them after each week.

Eventually they ran out of excuses and blocked my number, I know they did this because I called them from another trainer's phone and they answered, I just hung up, no point wasting any more of my time on these losers!

As a trainer, until you can figure out who is genuine and who isn't regarding this matter, you can find yourself hurting financially as you await a client's next session in which they're due to renew, but only to find they never actually show up leaving you without the money you're expecting to receive that you've already budgeted into your account. No big deal to them of course as they aren't the ones that are waiting for money to help pay bills, you are! This gets old very quickly and is very frustrating to say the least.

53

Of course it's my fault you're getting heavier!

Quite often as a trainer, you will be the one clients blame for not getting results, especially it seems regarding weight loss. Nothing to do with the fact they don't want to be accountable for what they're putting into their mouths of course! No, that would be too simple.

Any excuse is better than facing the truth, such as they believe you aren't training them correctly. Funny thing is, if they know better than you why are they paying you or any trainer good money to get in shape? Surely they could do it themselves and save a ton of money. After all, this isn't a cheap service so why waste money on something you aren't going to take seriously?

Get real people! You are paying a personal trainer to help you, but you won't allow yourself to be helped by constantly eating bad food, you don't have to be a brain surgeon to figure that one out!

One such issue arose when I trained Susan, she had contacted me wanting to lose weight but claiming she'd had 6 trainers over the last year but never got any results from any of them, if anything she'd gained weight! Now that's either some seriously bad trainers, or a client that won't do their part out of the gym by controlling what they're eating, with the chances of hiring 6 bad trainers back to back being very remote, I quickly figured out which reason it was, and equally as quickly figured she wasn't going to be an easy client to work with.

She was pleasant enough, but obviously had a love of unhealthy food. We worked out early Monday morning, and she would be telling me of how her weekend consisted of basically drinking beer and eating crappy food! Now, I warned her don't expect results from this if you're going to keep eating and drinking in that manner, she said she understood. I wasn't convinced in the slightest.

All was going well, she seemed to enjoy the workouts but when she stepped on the scales it was time for a reality check, she`d gained 5lb since the last weigh in 2 weeks before. Then of course it's time to blame the trainer "I think you're making me lift weights that are too heavy, I told you I didn't want to bulk up! We need to change the training program" she said like she's suddenly become an expert in personal training.

One thing I absolutely will not tolerate is having someone with no experience telling me I'm doing my job wrong! Delicate situation to handle though, on one hand I want to tell her she's stupid and to get lost! On the other hand this is a business so need to keep the money coming in. So I very politely reminded her of what she`d been telling me regarding what she`d been eating, and it wasn't healthy food by any means. Also explained to her to bulk someone up isn't as easy as she's thinking it was, that would require a very different training program than the one she was doing with me.

It became a regular battle every time she weighed in, unable to accept responsibility herself she would blame me for not training her correctly, and also reminding me of the thousands of dollars she had invested in my service. Realizing the sessions were over I figured it's time to put her in her place once and for all! I reminded her of the diet she was supposed to be on, but instead chose to eat crap food! As for the thousands of dollars, I told her she may as well have donated it to McDonalds! Which is basically what she did anyway.

She quit claiming she was going to find another trainer, one who knew what they were doing! Good luck on that. It was a relief when she walked out of the gym for the last time. So I guess I became the 7th bad trainer Susan had hired in a year. Oh well, I can live with that!

54

How many sessions do I have left? …None!

One issue that is particularly annoying is when clients cancel at the last minute, with excuses like "I can't make it today" or "I've been sick all day, can't make it" every so often things come up that are unavoidable like having to stay longer than expected at work, or a family member suddenly gets sick.

So occasionally it's a genuine reason, especially when it's an early morning client, after all anyone can wake up sick, not much you can do about that really. But mostly it's a lack of respect for your time, for example if someone has been sick all day and they cancel at the last minute they've had more than enough time to inform you, but for some reason chose not to, the reason being they simply don't care.

Personally, I experienced this kind of problem with evening clients, after a hard day's work not everyone feels like turning out again once they get home from work and start relaxing, or the weather might have turned bad since getting home. Understandable as it may be for not wanting to work out that particular night, you are at the gym waiting for them, you are keeping your end of the deal up, and they aren't.

Then of course you get the clients who simply don't bother to show up at all without informing you of anything! Chances are if you let them get away with it, then they'll keep doing it. As a trainer you'll get to know which clients pull this stunt regularly, and the quicker you put a stop to it the better it will be for you.

One such client was Maggie, she showed up claiming she was so serious about working out and never missed, just needed a few fresh ideas so decided to hire a trainer, that's fair enough, but by the looks of her she looked like she`d never missed a meal, not a training session!

She loved my style and paid for 20 sessions, she said it was just what she wanted and couldn't wait for the next session, funny thing was when the next session came around I was there, but Maggie wasn't. I called her and she told me her dog got loose earlier and she`d be there next session. With no thought of an apology for not showing up, this told me that this could possibly be an ongoing problem with Maggie.

That was to be the case unfortunately, one excuse after another, and on more than one occasion she actually admitted she had totally forgotten about having a training session with me. Kind of strange considering she was so serious about her workouts. Whatever!

As she had already signed to say she understood these sessions had to be used within 3 months, which is more than long enough for anyone to complete 20 sessions, and if she didn't show up without first informing me she`d lose the sessions. So I simply marked them off whether she was there or not, after all I was there, I hadn't forgotten she had a training session even if she had!

She came back a few times and we completed a total of 6 worthless sessions, after a while she just stopped making any excuses and not bothering to let me know anything at all. Her remaining 14 sessions were soon over with her not informing me she wasn't coming one single time!

Strangely enough a year later she emailed me saying she wanted a refund for the remaining 14 sessions! I quickly emailed her back a copy of the contract she signed knowing she had already lost those sessions. She never responded, nice try lady, but I had already covered my ass!

Good lesson here for any new trainers, make sure they understand they will be charged for the session if they don't show up with no warning, better still, actually get them to sign their name understanding that little issue before you even start training them. Many will complain about that claiming it's unfair, but how unfair was it when they decided to not come for their training session without even letting you know? After all, you made the effort to be there on time.

Again, if they know they can get away with it they'll keep doing it, and wasting your time, so nip it in the bud before it becomes a regular problem.

55

The old client who had a lot of old scores to settle!

Self-defense should not be about teaching you how to "go the distance" in a street fight or how to "teach someone a lesson" and certainly not about being a bully or attacking others when unprovoked. You are learning what to do in case you are attacked, how to gain that momentary edge over your attacker so you can get away or find people who can help you.

As self-defense and kickboxing have become a huge part of my personal training sessions it was no surprise when I received an email from a guy requesting self-defense training. This time though the client had sinister reasons for wanting to learn these skills!

Chester showed up for his first training session, complete with back, knee, shoulder and elbow problems! So teaching someone self-defense with these issues is pretty difficult, if it's just to learn out on interest, or for fun, then fine, but when you consider the speed these moves have to be performed at to be effective, then any hope of using them to truly protect yourself with is pretty slim really. But he said he always wanted to learn self-defense out of interest and use as exercise, so that's fair enough and we set about teaching him the basics first.

Well without sounding rude, this guy was incredibly slow on his feet, and at 67 why wouldn't he be? But for exercise it would work fine. After a few minutes he started asking questions like "What move would work best if I wanted to really teach someone a lesson?" I tried to explain that's not the idea behind self-defense, and there's no way I could possibly answer that simply because you can't say what you would do if attacked, once the adrenalin kicks in and takes over then anything could happen, also certain moves would work better than others depending on the angle you were being attacked from. He said he understood but still continued to ask me similar questions regularly.

Nearly every session Chester made several references to two old classic movies, namely Dirty Harry with Clint Eastwood and Deathwish with Charles Bronson, which actually happened to be two of my all-time favorite movies so was more than happy to discuss the action scenes with him and relive these classic movies, and it certainly helped make the hours training session go by very fast. As these movies were about getting the bad guys, there's a common theme here, and it got me thinking…

I started to realize this guy wasn't thinking of using these moves as self-defense, but rather using them to attack someone! Out of curiosity I asked him exactly why he really wanted to know these things. He then went into great detail about a school reunion coming up next year that he needed to be prepared for. Apparently he had several scores to settle, and that was his real reason behind wanting to learn these moves.

Now this is a really crazy situation, this guy has held a grudge against so many people, some for over 50 years! He had a list of names, and went into great detail about who did what to him and what year it happened. Now he plans to teach them all a lesson during a school reunion! Slight problem though, he's so slow if he ever tries to use these moves for real they'll see it coming long before he even gets close to doing any of them!

Thankfully though, it seems he was just venting and liked to talk tough, he stayed training with me for almost a year, actually leading up to the school reunion, then strangely enough, never even went to it! I guess he realized he had no chance of pulling this off even if he was serious which I don't think he ever really was, as he never got any faster at all!

He quit soon after saying his injuries prevented him from getting revenge on all these people from the past, but the next school reunion they'd better watch out! He claimed he'd be back in training for that. As that was another five years away I didn't get too excited about the chances of training him again. Quite a character though that's for sure.

56

A ghost was seen in the gym… Maybe!

One of the very first gyms I worked at years ago was rumored to have been actually built on an old grave yard, I don't know if this is true or not but can remember the whole area years before being a little spooky, before they started to develop it when it was nothing more than waste land and a large dumping ground. Firstly they built a nightclub that failed after a couple of years, then came the gym which was a great success.

Anyway, several people reported sightings of an old man dressed in old fashioned clothes walking through the gym late at night. I never thought anything much about this until one night I was heading back to the gym for my last client of the night, where upon arrival I found another trainer totally freaking out, he was completely white and shaking!

I said "What's up? You look like you've just seen a ghost!" which of course freaked him out even more as apparently that's exactly what he had just seen! After several minutes he calmed down enough to tell me he saw this old man and thinking it was a potential client who wandered into the gym (this did happen occasionally) went to see if he could assist this man, he said he followed him around the corner where the man vanished before his very own eyes!

I know this sounds crazy, and actually my first reaction was to laugh, but as this was a very level headed type of guy who was obviously very distressed, I didn't. He was so freaked out that he actually ran out of the gym, and quit the job claiming he could never go back in that gym ever again! He was convinced he really had seen a ghost! He was a good trainer, and despite many people's attempts at trying to talk him into reconsidering his decision, he never did come back.

It was kind of a spooky feeling in there at night afterwards for a while knowing whatever it was he saw made him quit and never want to come back ever again. What really happened I don't know, but I found myself now listening to every little noise in that gym. However, no one ever saw the mysterious man or ghost or whatever it was ever again. So it was all forgotten about pretty quickly. The trainer in question seemed to vanish as no one else heard from or saw him again for a long time after that.

Around two years later I came across that same trainer once again when I was out with friends one night, we were reliving old stories and of course I brought up that particular night he saw the ghost. He admitted as he was feeling under a lot of stress from work and home he had been taking magic mushrooms, anyway that night he took too many and was hallucinating and actually went on to have a complete breakdown! We both had a really good laugh about this now the truth was finally revealed.

A ghost in the gym?...I think not!

57

After hours cardio session with a difference!

As it was company policy that no one person alone was allowed to lock up the gym at the end of each night, there always had to be two people for security reasons, this particular night It was my turn, and I had the job of staying late with the fitness manager, we locked up at the usual time and went home. Nothing unusual at this stage, just the end of another typical night in the gym.

When I left the gym I went to a friend's house for a couple of hours first. On my way home I needed to use the toilet but it was past 11.00pm so knew the pubs would be closed so I couldn't stop there. As I was passing the gym where I worked I thought I'll go behind it as it overlooked a large wasteland area.

On my way up the drive I noticed the light was on in the manager's office, strange I thought as only two hours previously I had help lock up so knew everyone had left for the night, anyway after doing my business behind the gym I saw a car I recognized parked behind a dumpster, something didn't seem quite right here so I thought I would investigate.

After quietly approaching the office window I could hear groaning noises from inside so very carefully I peeked in. To my amazement I saw the fitness manager and a female trainer totally naked on top of the managers desk screwing like there were no tomorrow! Both were married, but not to one another! As the girl had a great body I thought I would watch a while longer but accidentally kicked over a coke can someone had conveniently left by my feet!

Shit! Both of them heard this and looked straight at the window just missing seeing my grinning face admiring their afterhours work! Time to get out of there fast. I quickly ran to my car and drove off at high speed with the lights off so they would have no idea what make of car they were looking at, if indeed they had even bothered to look.

Next morning at the gym I told someone, who told someone else and they told someone else and so on and so on…basically, after the first hour everyone in the gym knew about what had happened the night before, people were getting called in the office one after another as they tried to trace the original source of the gossip.

By the time they had narrowed it down to me, both the assistant manager and the female trainer had both been suspended. When it was my turn to be interrogated I was greeted in the office by three people from head office all of whom were very serious looking and obviously meant business.

The whole thing was ridiculous. The first hour was spent explaining why I was using the back of the gym as a toilet! How much simpler could It be? I needed to piss and was passing by! After three hours I was released, they took a five page statement from me which resulted in both the fitness manager and female trainer getting fired.

A few years later, I bumped into the former fitness manager in a local pub who was now running his own successful personal training business, we got talking about old times and he said "Best thing that ever happened getting fired from that place, pity I don't know who did it as I'd buy them a drink" with a huge grin on my face I said "it was me, and I'll have a pint thanks!"

58

Crazy scenes behind the gym during our lunch!

During the summertime a few other trainers and myself would try and time it right that we didn't have clients at a certain time on Fridays so we could enjoy having lunch together outside at the back of the gym, it was impossible to do this every day, but Friday we usually managed it. It was a nice setting with a small river running down below, and it got us out of the sweaty gym for an hour in the fresh air, well it wasn't so fresh this particular day though.

The next building behind the gym and across the river happened to be the local slaughter house, so plenty of squealing coming from that direction this day and most days recently. I think they were receiving a good supply of pigs this particular summer. The squeals and smell were a little too much for many people who had quickly lost their appetite and chose to return back inside the gym to finish their lunch. They missed quite a day.

Half way through the lunch hour a breeze picked up and the smell of the slaughter house was brought right to our nostrils! The squeals were one thing but the smell of pigs being slaughtered was something else, we decided to all go back inside as it was getting too much for us now, even the guys with the strongest stomachs were feeling it.

All of a sudden the squeals got louder and louder. We were amazed to see a pig charging down the side of the gym towards us! Naturally we all cheered the pig on, the pig had escaped but only had a few minutes of freedom as the workers from the slaughter house caught up with him and quickly returned the pig back to meet his maker! Nice try pig, but not your lucky day after all, ten out of ten for effort though!

As we were gathering up our lunches we noticed what looked like a body floating past down in the river below! We immediately thought it was some kind of dummy and weren't too concerned about it really. It was too far away to see clearly, but looked too rigid to be real. So we continued to gather up our lunches and head back inside.

Next thing we know a bunch of police officers came running around the top of the river bank claiming someone had jumped off the bridge in the local park about a mile away. They said they were looking for a body, I pointed over to my left and said "I think it went that way" they told us we might want to go back inside at this point and quickly disappeared down the river bank to retrieve the body.

We figured that was probably good advice, but with the excitement starting to build, we chose to ignore their advice and hung around a bit longer, and soon wishing we hadn't as five minutes later they came back up the river bank dragging a dead body with them! This was where we all lost our lunches. By this time the police were everywhere and sealed off the area behind the gym. All afternoon and into the evening more and more police kept on coming and turned the whole area into a crime scene.

What with all the drama of police everywhere, the smell of pigs being slaughtered, the runaway pig and the sight of a dead body it wasn't a very pleasant lunch hour that day, exciting for sure though. That was the end of our summer lunchtimes outside, from then on we stayed inside the gym instead, and the smell of the sweaty gym didn't seem to bother anyone anymore after that incident!

59

The secret fire drill in the gym, every man for himself!

This particular day the gym manager had arranged a secret fire drill with the local fire department. Secret because they wanted to observe the staff and trainers dealing with the sudden threat of a fire and leading the gym members and clients out to safety, many plain clothes firemen were there working out acting like members to observe our reaction.

We had many fire drills before but always pre-arranged so it was no big deal really, just the usual procedure of making your way to the nearest exit and calmly leading anyone in the gym outside in an orderly manner, and as there were so many exits it was a very easy task. This day however, was to be very different and a total disaster, well, at least according to the under-cover firemen, not me!

The main gym floor and large cardio room were separated by big blue heavy plastic strip curtains similar to the ones found in warehouses. Anyway, a few of the plain clothes firemen had positioned themselves outside this area to see the reaction of the staff.

As the alarm sounded I happened to be heading back from the storage room carrying a big box of protein drinks over my shoulder heading towards the reception area via the gym floor, I shouted "Shit! Fire!" I very quickly dropped the box I was carrying and charged full speed through the curtains knocking a fireman off his feet in the process! Kicked open the nearest exit and ran to the area of the car park designated for fire drills, all in all I was very impressed by my quick thinking actions, unfortunately no one else was!

The gym manager was furious and said the fire chief would be coming to talk with me about my actions this day. Indeed most of the staff had fled the building in total panic forgetting about anyone else still inside, only the management came to the rescue of the members who ignored the alarm, then again only the management knew this was going to happen, so had a slight advantage over the rest of us.

The fire chief told me I was a disgrace and should be ashamed of myself! I took an instant disliking to this guy and proceeded to tell him I certainly was not going to play the hero and put my life in danger running around the gym looking for people still working out while a fire was happening in there! Oh, and I also told him he chose that job as a fireman and was getting paid a hell of a lot more than me to put his life in danger! That told him!

I was told I would have to take special training focusing on protecting the precious public. No problem I thought, I'll take all the special training you want but if a fire really happens I'm still no fireman, and I'll get myself out of there as fast as possible first every time....Every man for himself!

60

Let's add a move... then break my own arm!

Stress these days is a major problem, and I see that with so many of my clients when they come to the gym. It's a very satisfying feeling when they leave after one hour in a much better frame of mind than when they arrived. That's why my kickboxing training really helps with this issue.

Punching a bag after a frustrating day at work is certainly a great stress reliever. To actually feel the contact of your punches against a solid object will feel more realistic and put you in a better frame of mind should you be stressed out that day, as many clients particularly with office jobs seem to be these days.

You just can't pretend to punch like shadow boxing, that won't do anything at all to relieve stress, you need feedback and by visualizing the punching bag as a symbol that was the source of your stress and aggravation for the day as you pound it with punches is a much more productive method than using negative ways of relieving stress such as getting physical with someone. Relieving stress in a negative manner simply leads to more stress sooner or later.

My punching bags quite often get named after client's bosses or even their husbands or wives! A punching bag will allow you to express and release your frustrations, and ultimately relieve your stress without getting yourself into trouble or hurt. Now, having said all that, as you're striking a solid object in the form of a punching bag care must be taken when delivering punches and kicks, as one misplaced punch could spell disaster, as it did for a particular client of mine one night.

Michael had been coming to me for training a few years with great results, but when he had a new boss at work who he claimed didn't like him, he really stepped up the kickboxing and named the punching bags after his new boss, which certainly helped keep the workouts lively, until one night he took it a step too far…

This particular night we were practicing temple strikes with a back fist which involved nothing more than stepping forward and delivering a blow with the back of the fist, pretty simple stuff really, but when performed at very high speed in a non-stop fashion for 2 minutes it can become very challenging.

Michael had got this down to perfection, and with the adrenalin pumping big time he started shouting out his bosses name with every strike! Then for some reason he suddenly performed a spinning back fist strike which he totally miss-timed, and with the speed of his movement there was a sickening crack as he delivered his blow, sadly though with his elbow and not his fist.

"I think I just broke my arm" he said, I'm thinking I know you've just broken your arm! That unmistakable cracking sound was pretty obvious what had happened. He sat the rest of the session out and left feeling very sorry for himself.

A trip to the hospital confirmed his arm was indeed broken, he was out for a couple of weeks, but returned and did the treadmill until he felt comfortable enough to try kickboxing once again.

61

The sex crazed and foul-mouthed female client!

One thing for sure about this job is you really do meet some very colorful characters to say the least! But every once in a while you come across the kind of client who is totally oblivious to anyone else being in the gym while they loudly broadcast their private lives for all to hear in graphic detail, and understandably of course not everyone appreciates hearing such things. There's a reason it's called a private life, private as in keep it to yourself!

The first time it was kind of funny, but when it became every session it was less funny each time and soon got very old. The client in question here was Jessica, a small young lady believed to be from somewhere in the middle east but no one really knew for sure, and strangely enough, not even Jessica herself!

I first met Jessica a year ago when she called me claiming she needed to firm up a little, but otherwise was happy with her appearance. So I'm thinking this shouldn't be too difficult really. The first session was unbelievable! The gym was packed with clients, many who happened to be elderly. Jessica was on the leg extension when she suddenly shouted out "My fucking pussy is sore as shit!" while rubbing herself at the same time.

Now that really got everyone's attention, with most people not quite sure if they had just heard that little outburst correctly. Just so there was no misunderstandings, Jessica shouted out "I knew I shouldn't have fucked those two guys together last night!" Ok, a little too much information there young lady.

The expressions on the faces of the elderly people-many of which were big church going people-was one of pure shock and horror, not to mention disgust! During the session there were several similar outbursts from Jessica, but she saved the best, or worst depending on how you view this till last. I had her performing ab exercises when the Marvin Gaye song `Sexual Healing` came on the radio, her sit ups suddenly became simulated sex! She was now writhing on the floor singing along and shouting "Oh yes, fuck me harder!" Some found it amusing, but most were in total shock. For me personally, I found it difficult to understand why she was so oblivious to so many other people being in the gym around her. I mean, it's one thing to be an exhibitionist, but this was way over the top.

Of course after this session many people complained to me about Jessica`s behavior, many stating they didn't feel comfortable around that kind of vulgar talk. But what am I supposed to do about it? Like her or not, she's a paying client. Get over it people! I agreed to have a word with her, not that it would do any good as I'd tried that several times before with no results. Jessica said they'll get over it, they need to liven up a bit!

Interestingly enough, the next session the gym was completely empty, but nothing changed as Jessica gave a repeat performance of her exploits in graphic detail once again as only she could! This puzzled me, as there was no one else around to hear her stories so why even bother telling them in such detail, not to mention telling them so loudly? I quickly came to the conclusion she was just plain nuts! No other description for her really.

The next session the gym was packed again, this should be interesting I'm thinking to myself. We hadn't even got through the warm up before Jessica started with her stories once again! "I got fucked last night so hard my legs are wobbling!" she shouted out loudly for all to hear. Next up was walking lunges where she stopped every few seconds to rub herself shouting out "My pussy is really fucking sore today!" The whole session was like that and for the next two weeks it was the same until one day she told me she was going to have to quit training, much to the relief of the majority of the gym of course. This was her exact graphic explanation, all told in her usual loud and vulgar way of course so everyone else in the gym could hear every word.

"I can`t train anymore because I'm getting married, I've only known this guy two weeks and I'm pregnant, not sure who the father is, could be one of the six or seven guys I've fucked recently, no idea really"

So that was the end of Jessica in the gym, and to be honest I wasn't too disappointed as all the drama was getting a little too much. No idea whatever happened to her until one day a few years later I saw her in a local store, she was walking around with two kids and a third on the way! I actually heard her before I saw her as she was swearing and carrying on in her own unique vulgar way. Not too impressive sounding either in front of little kids. I quickly disappeared before she saw me as I had no interest in hearing what she'd been doing since our last training session.

The evidence was there for all to see, two kids and a third one on the way! She had been very busy indeed, no wonder she hadn't been back to the gym, and we`re all quite thankful for that!

62

The kid that thought video game fighting was realistic!

One of the most popular training sessions I offer is self-defense, and people have many reasons for wanting to learn this, most of course wish to learn this to protect themselves. But when someone wants to learn it because of what they've seen on video games, and then doesn't even think it's realistic you could say they're a little confused as they cannot separate make believe from reality.

One such client was a 14 year old kid who had persuaded his parents to buy him self-defense sessions after becoming obsessed with it after playing these fighting video games. However, my realistic style of self-defense didn't quite live up to his unrealistic expectations.

He started asking questions like how could he rip someone's spine out like he's seen on his video games! When I told him that was just in video games and not even possible he claimed I said that because I didn't know how to do that particular move! So I quickly figured these sessions were not going to be easy at all.

The kid was totally obsessed by these video games, especially the fighting ones. Surely at 14 years of age he should know they're not real…shouldn't he? Maybe a kid at 8 years old could be forgiven for being confused, but at 14, come on now! Let's get real here.

The next session I'm trying to teach him how to escape from being grabbed from behind, but he has other ideas! This session he wants to learn how to rip someone's heart out and show it them before they die! Again, I tell him that's not possible and try to explain what he's seeing on his video games is not possible in real life. Once again, he accuses me of not knowing how to perform this particular move, and it went on like this for several sessions.

Ok, time for a reality check here. I've had enough of this nonsense and call the parents. They tell me they're so happy he's coming to me for self-defense and he talks about your sessions all the time! Really? We haven't even done a self-defense session yet, all we`ve done is listen to this kid talk nonsense about the crap he's seen playing video games.

To my amazement they renew at an even bigger package than the first one! Well, I guess money is money and if they don't mind wasting it then I'll take it! The sessions carry on much the same as before with the kid trying to re-live everything he's been playing thinking it`s real. Then he starts to tell his parents that I'm teaching him all these crazy moves from the video games, which isn't true. Not a good situation developing here.

The parents call wanting to know why I'm not teaching him real self-defense instead of what he's seeing on video games. They go into great detail about how the fighting on his video games isn't actually real! Really? No shit! I tell them instead of telling me I suggest they tell their son as I know they're not real, he doesn't! And while we`re at it, why are they letting him play these things so much leaving him with a totally warped sense of reality.

They claim the video games are just harmless fun and it keeps him busy instead of running the streets at night. Harmless fun? I don't think so, not when he thinks they're real. Anyway, thankfully they pulled him out of our training sessions once the current package was over and I was quite happy to see the back of him!

Now, I'm not saying video games are bad, but like everything else they must be played in moderation.

What we had here was simply a case of a young kid being allowed to play video games to the point of it being an obsession where the make believe had become reality to him. Seems like the parents let him play them so much as it kept him occupied and out of their hair! An all too familiar story in this fast paced modern technology age we find ourselves in. Video games and cell phones are turning the kids of today into zombies!

63

Smoking at the gym doors seconds before a training session!…Really?

Everyone knows smoking and exercising don't go together right? But when someone is so addicted they just have to have that last smoke right before entering the gym, then you know they have a serious problem, and most likely won't have the energy to last the full hour no matter how bad they claim to want results, it's just not going to happen.

Steve was such a client, he had contacted me asking for help to bulk up a little, he was 6'5" and weighed in at 160lb, and in his own words he was like a walking tooth pick! My first thought was from hearing those details of his height and weight this sounded like an accurate description without even seeing him. He was getting married in 6 months so wanted to put a little size on. He also told me he smoked like crazy and ate very little. As he worked in a local foundry he was burning off way more calories than he was consuming.

So all in all, we have our work cut out here I'm thinking if we're going to get the results he wishes. The smoking, lack of food and the hard physical job are not in his favor, so many changes needed here! But he seemed like a genuinely nice guy, and as I'm always up for a challenge I agreed to take him on, he signed up for 20 sessions and we arranged the first training session.

I happened to be looking out of the gym window when Steve pulled up in his truck, he was early so sat there smoking for 10 minutes! Hardly ideal preparation I'm thinking. As if that wasn't bad enough, he walked over to the entrance of the gym and stood by the door and finished smoking his cigarette! Ok that's a new one for me, never seen that before.

When he came in we started off on the treadmill for a 5 minute warm up at a very steady pace, he was struggling big time! Stinking of cigarettes, and pouring with sweat he was dead on his feet after the 5 minutes claiming he was so unfit he needed to sit down a few minutes. 10 minutes later he had recovered enough to start the training session.

Needless to say, it was a very slow paced first session as I tried to observe his strengths and weaknesses, plenty of weaknesses and no strengths at this stage it seemed! As he was so skinny I told him he could get away with eating way more food, and really needed to especially with the job he's doing. He needs the extra fuel just to get through the shift, let alone the training session and of course cut back on the smoking, as at present that's the biggest problem as it's cutting his appetite down considerably.

He tried his best with the weights but just didn't have the energy or strength to succeed. We completed 8 sessions of the 20 he had paid for when he quit saying the training was way too hard on his body! He also claimed the training was making his body too sore to do his job properly. Every session he continued to show up smoking and also smoking right up till he walked in the gym.

He thanked me for trying to help him but he admitted it was his fault it wasn't working and was never likely to work because he couldn't give up his excessive smoking habit. As a gesture of goodwill he said keep the money as he was sorry for wasting my time. I didn't bother to remind him he had already signed stating he would lose the sessions if he didn't use them, so I already knew that I was keeping the money! But I thanked him anyway. That was the last I saw of him, hopefully he managed to cut back on the smoking, but probably not I'm thinking.

Still to this day, I have never seen anyone stand at the gym doors smoking seconds before starting a training session! How could he seriously claim to expect results with this kind of preparation? Some people really haven't a clue. Sadly Steve was one of those, nice guy, but totally clueless!

64

The parents who followed the kid around the gym…No pressure!

One of the most annoying and irritating situations I've come across doing this job is when you get parents bringing their kids along and follow the kids every move around the gym giving what they think is encouragement, but actually putting the kid under so much pressure they can't relax and enjoy the training session. It's one thing to show interest, and quite natural to do so, but this goes way beyond that.

A couple emailed me saying their 13 year old kid was being bullied at school and wanted to hire a trainer during the summer holiday to beef him up a little and show him a few self-defense techniques in order to defend himself once he returned back to school. Seems like a fair enough request I'm thinking, so we arranged a time for them to visit the gym and look around.

When they arrived it was obvious the parents were going to do all the talking and never actually gave the kid chance to speak for himself. He was already a very skinny, shy kid and very intimidated by the whole thing. But I figured once we got the training sessions under way I'd be able to bring the kid from out of his shell so to speak. Unfortunately, that was to prove very difficult with his parents.

They brought him for his first session and to my surprise stayed around for the warm up. Ok I'm thinking, they'll leave anytime now so I can work on this kid's insecurity. Not only did they stay for the warm up, but chose to stay the whole session following us around the gym watching his every move, and giving him advice on what he should be doing like "You can lift more than that son!" and "Put more effort in son!" I thought that's what they're paying me for isn't it? Worse than that was the fact both parents were very overweight. This went on for the first 3 sessions. I could clearly see the kid was hating it and couldn't relax. This wasn't going to work at all.

So I called them and explained the situation as I saw it, I asked them to give me 5 sessions alone with the kid to help him relax as this would be beneficial to everyone concerned, not least of all…me! My plan worked and the kid instantly felt the pressure lift from his shoulders and actually began to enjoy his training sessions and made some good gains in size, strength and more importantly his confidence. Under the shyness was a nice intelligent kid that respected what I was trying to achieve for him. We made a good team and powered through the workouts with great success.

His parents were delighted with their `new look` kid and agreed it was the best move they made by staying away from the training sessions, they dropped him off, then came and picked him back up an hour later. Everyone happy, they continued to pay for his training sessions the whole of the school holidays, and kept in regular touch after he returned to school telling me no one could believe the changes in this kids body and mind. Thankfully there were no more reports of him being bullied. Don't you just love a story with a happy ending?

Seriously though parents, when you pay for your kids training sessions you really don't have to follow them around the gym and watch their every move, it's very discouraging for the kid, and for the trainer for that matter. Just leave them with the trainer for the hour, and like the kid in this story I'm sure you'll all benefit from doing so.

65

Shoplifters in the gym? That's different!

One of the first gyms I ever worked at was without doubt one of the strangest, if not the strangest I've ever seen let alone worked at! The gym manager didn't even workout himself, and had no interest in doing so, he owned several successful businesses, and claimed this was the future for gyms, but clearly didn't understand the concept of how a gym should look. As this gym was located in a not so nice area of town it attracted the not so nice people. Shoplifting was soon to be a regular problem.

As you entered the gym the very first thing you saw even before the reception was a little area almost like a corner store that sold everything from candy to soda etc. His theory was why not sell everything to make extra money, once word got around it actually worked as it became very busy with people choosing to buy their junk food from the gym rather than the corner store, mainly because he was undercutting the local corner stores, who were seriously not happy! Good business it seemed, but junk food in a gym? Just something about that doesn't seem right somehow.

Part of my duties as a personal trainer in this crazy gym-apart from training people-was to unload trucks bringing in all this crap, stock the shelves and manage endless amounts of worthless paperwork! Plus chase shoplifters all over town until we caught them, at least that was the gym manager's theory but certainly not mine, or anyone else's that worked there!

As I was getting paid a really crap wage and working crazy hours I certainly wasn't going to play the hero by putting myself at risk by tackling some crazy shoplifter, there had already been several instances of shoplifters beating and even stabbing the gym staff! The gym manager was too tight to pay for official security but expected us to do it. My way of thinking was if they could get away with stealing something…good luck to them! I certainly wasn't going to lose any sleep over it!

That being said, it still didn't stop us from having some fun chasing them though, at least until we were out of sight of the gym then run into the nearest pub, have a quick pint, then go back to the gym telling them we had chased them into the town center but couldn't catch them as they had a friend in a car waiting to pick them up.

The gym manager would fall for it every time and would actually give us gift certificates in thanks for our help! It got us out of that crazy place for an hour, get a pint and return empty handed and get rewarded, this happened so many times, but he never stopped to think why we never actually caught anyone...ever!

It was quite a regular occurrence to hear the girl on reception put the call out of "Staff announcement, code 51" which was our secret code to say get ready someone's about to do a runner, or already taken off with stolen goods. So we were expected to drop everything and chase after them and bring back the precious goods they had stolen....Whatever!

On this particular occasion a young kid of about 16 had stolen a few packs of cigarettes and made it out of the gym, so me and two of my work friends were in hot pursuit straight across the parking lot heading towards the town center, the kid was crapping himself as he couldn't out run us, we always gave them a head start as we had no intentions of catching them so always made sure we were out of sight of the gym before we eased off, this is where the kid stopped and looking shit scared, holding his hands up and out of breath saying "Ok you got me I give in, here's the cigarettes I stole, I'm sorry"

We ran straight past him laughing and kept on running up the road to the nearest pub! I always remember looking back and seeing this kid flying back down the road like the devil was after him! Within seconds he had got his second wind going from exhaustion to shock! He couldn't believe his luck that day.

This was a regular occurrence in that gym, and it carried on like that for another 3 months, then thankfully the gym manager sold the business to someone else, who of course immediately closed down the little store, much to the relief of us, not to mention the local corner stores and attempted to make the gym look like a proper gym as it should have been in the first place. No more junk food sold in that gym!

Funny thing was, the old gym manager always told us he would open a chain of these new style gyms saying "Mark my words, this is the future of gyms" well, thankfully that wasn't the case.

SUCCESS STORIES

The last part of my book is proof that it's not all been about strange experiences in the gym, or training crazy people over the years who aren't taking their training seriously. Many times clients come along who are very serious about their training and get great results when they listen and follow my advice.

Here's a few testimonials from clients who achieved their fitness goals, and in particular lost weight, a lot of weight! Knowing you have given your client exactly what they wanted and paid for, and made their life healthier is the most rewarding feeling for a personal trainer.

So results can be achieved when a trainer and client both do their part. It really is a team effort, and quite simply one won't work without the other. These testimonials can be seen on my website **www.britwillgetufit.com**

Lisa Perez – Lost 65lbs!

I knew I needed help losing weight, I had tried every diet there is, but nothing really worked for me. So my doctor advised me to seek the help of a personal trainer. I stumbled across Nigel as I waded through the endless ads for trainers, with apprehension I signed up for a few sessions. To my amazement I actually liked it as it was just what I was looking for. Nigel was the answer to my problems with his unique training style and sense of humor that made working out fun, but also hard work! He somehow made me enjoy getting my butt kicked! Trust me, this guy will get you in shape, just wish I`d have found him before I wasted all that money on those stupid diets! But better late than never and I`m enjoying my new look 65lbs lighter. Thank you Nigel.

Adam Carter – Lost 120lbs!

My last remaining option before gastric bypass surgery was sign up with a personal trainer, everything else had failed so I thought why not? I really didn't want the surgery and neither did my doctor. So I signed up with Nigel, who I instantly felt was on my side and not just in it for the money, which was important as this is by no means a cheap service! But what price is your health? I mean, if I didn't do this I`d be spending a fortune on medical bills in later life.

I`m not going to lie, the training felt like hell to start with! but with Nigel`s encouragement and excellent training methods he kept me focused and I soon started feeling better about myself, then the weight started coming off. In just under 2 years I have lost 120lbs! I have never felt better in my life.

In Nigel, I haven't just found a trainer, but also a good friend who has taught me how to really change my lifestyle totally! I`m now learning and enjoying kick boxing, something I never thought was possible for me to do.

I would recommend Nigel in a heartbeat...Nigel, you're the best!

Debbie Haynes – Lost 190lbs!

Ok, so first things first, I knew when I got into this that it wasn't going to be easy or quick. I knew my trainer had to be someone special that could not only handle the job required, but also deal with my frustrations and lack of patience! I`m glad to say Nigel met all the requirements needed, he never gave up on me when I was ready to quit many times, the early days were very rough indeed. But with Nigel`s help I kept on track.

Every workout seemed to be so different, so there was never a chance of getting bored. As Nigel had warned me the diet side of things would be the hardest and he wasn't joking either! it was pure hell! But here I am now, almost 200lbs lighter, without resorting to surgery.

I consider myself living proof of the fact that if you really want something bad enough, you can actually get it! I know I could never have achieved the results I did without Nigel. If you are serious about getting in shape, then you must hire this guy as the results speak for themselves!

Chris Simms – Lost 45lbs!

Having been the victim of an unprovoked attack a few years ago, I wanted to learn how to defend myself, apart from wanting to lose quite a bit of weight of course. Slight problem trying to come up with the money to hire a personal trainer and also a self-defense instructor.

I had tried a few trainers that were ok, but didn't really offer what I wanted, sorry guys, but a few punches on the hand pads does not pass as kickboxing training! I wanted more than that, but couldn't find it.

So, Enter Nigel Taylor, a personal trainer who does everything from weights and kickboxing to self-defense! I`m glad to say this trainer can back his words up. With Nigel`s help I have not only lost weight, but, also learned how to defend myself too, all while having a blast! This guy is funny as hell!

I feel like I have come a long way, both physically and mentally since I started my journey to get in shape. With Nigel`s unique blend of multiple styles that cover everything, and believe me he really does cover everything! I have achieved a look and confidence I never thought possible, can you imagine how lucky I feel to have met this guy? Thank you Nigel.

Meet the author

Nigel Taylor, Originally from Chesterfield-a small market town in the north of England-exchanged the rain and cold weather of his homeland for the sunshine and heat of south Texas back in 2001 where he's lived ever since and operates his own successful personal training business specializing in kick boxing and self-defense based out of Round Rock Texas, where he now lives with his beautiful fiancé soon to be wife Stormy, and crazy dog Charlie Taylor who resembles Scooby Doo!

Taylor a world traveler, first got the travel bug when he visited Barbados back in 1988, followed by trips to India, Pakistan, Mexico, Cancun, Jamaica, Florida, Las Vegas, Cuba, Japan, Dubai, Kuwait, Bahrain, Costa Rica, Greece, Spain, Portugal, France, Holland, Belgium, Denmark, Sweden, Switzerland, Austria, Germany, Balearic Islands, Canary Islands and last but not least Thailand which soon became Taylor`s favorite destination visiting this paradise in Southeast Asia on numerous occasions studying Thai boxing. His many visits enabling a touch of realism to be added to his writing on this exotic and fascinating destination.

Other books available by Nigel Taylor
www.britaintowritten.com

Fitness & Fun
Confusion in Pattaya
Danger in Pattaya
The rise and fall of a gym owner
The crazy world of online dating
The crazy world of online dating – Part 2

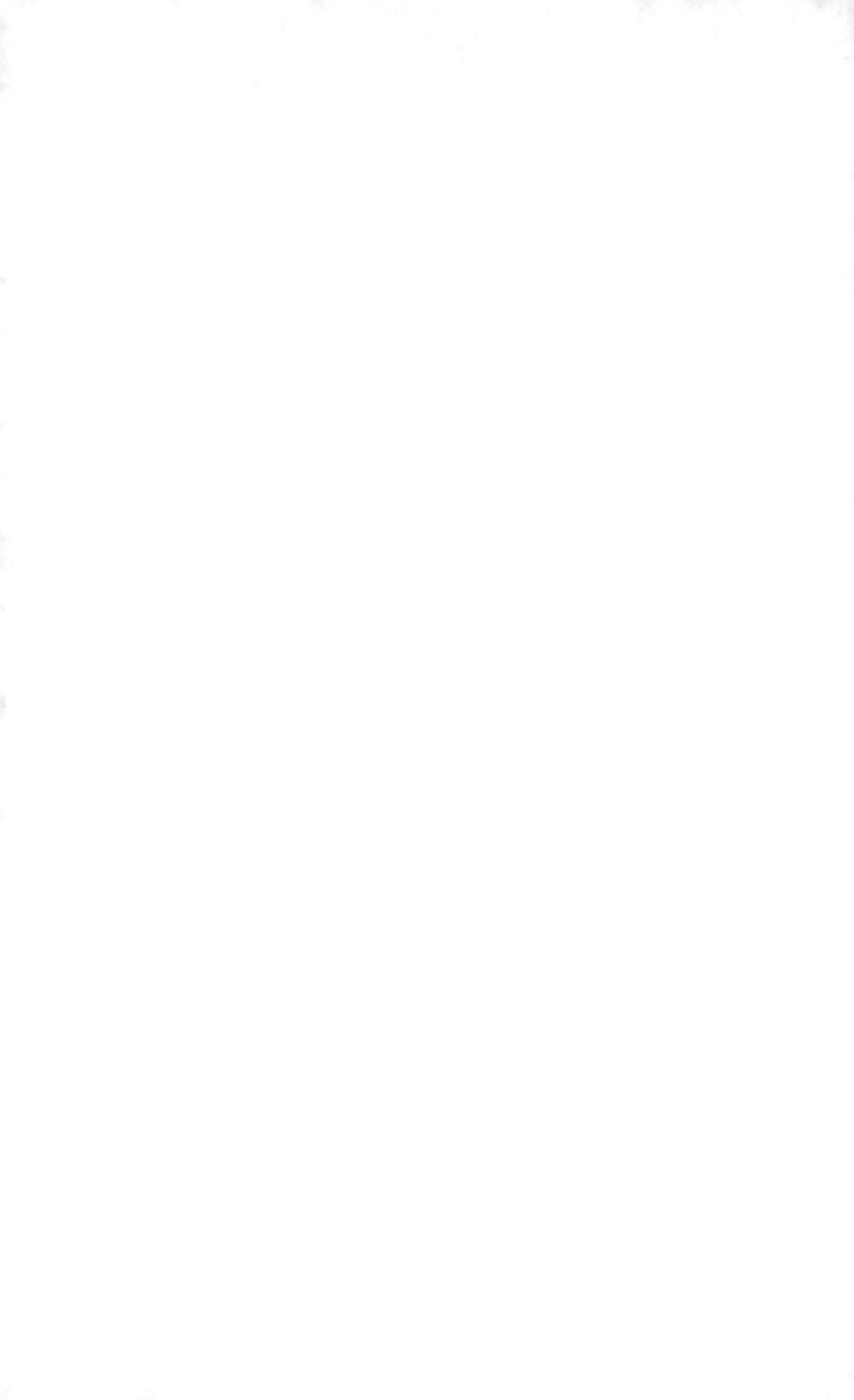

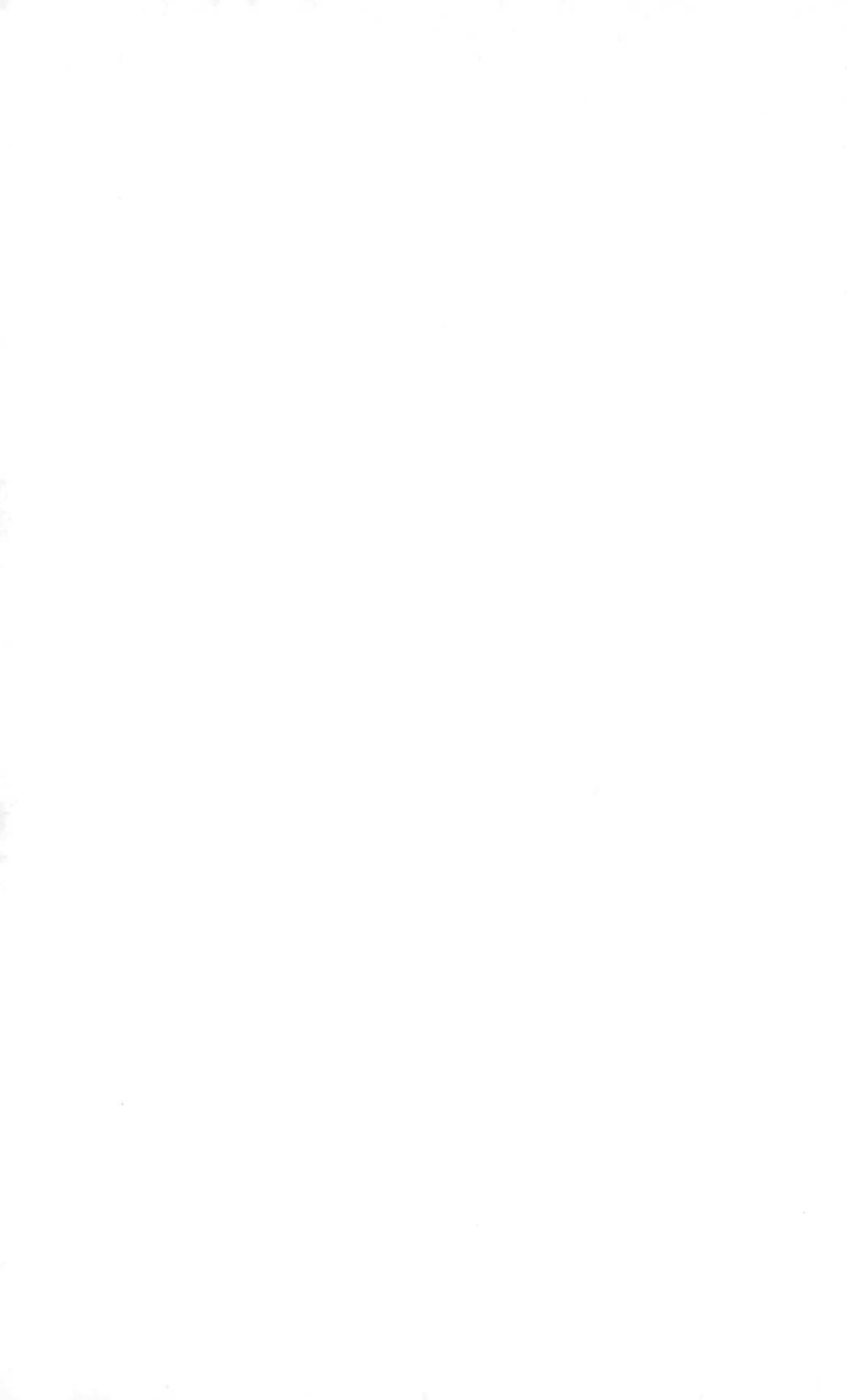

www.ingramcontent.com/pod-product-compliance
Lightning Source LLC
Chambersburg PA
CBHW070852290526
45795CB00001B/94